Table of Contents

FOREWORD

This is a story of the beginning of stroke recovery. On September 7, 2016, I suffered a moderate stroke that completely paralyzed my left side. This is my effort to chronicle the early stages of my recovery and my wholehearted attempt to defeat this stroke and fully recover to being "normal." First a little bit about me.

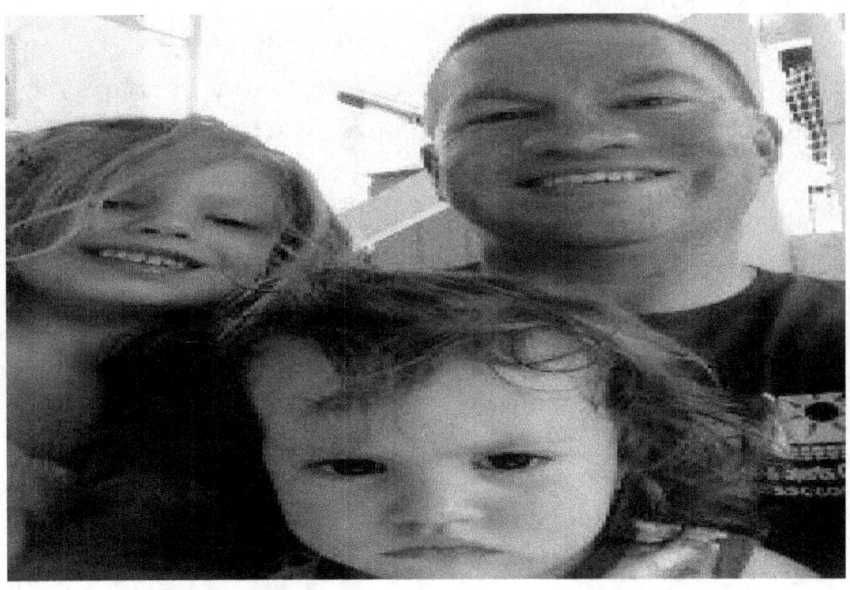

An older picture of me and my girls

I'm a 49-year-old man with 6-and10-year-old girls. I am happily married to a wonderful woman who will be part of this chronicle.

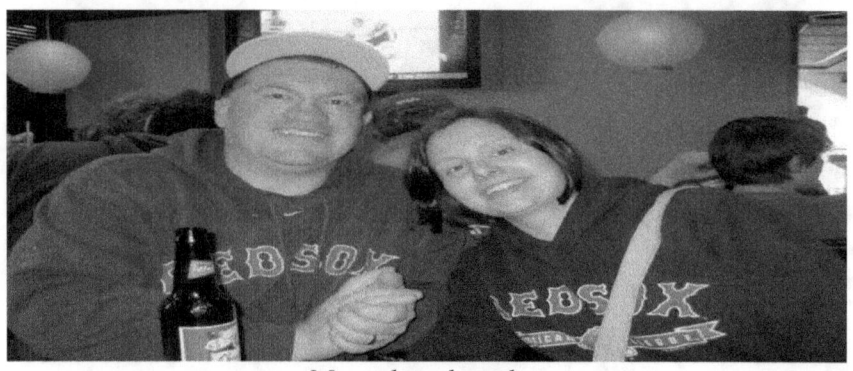
Me and my broad

I work for the state department of education in Massachusetts mostly working with high school improvement including dropout prevention. I'm happy to say I love my work and, as I realize now had a perfect life until the evening of September 7. I live in Melrose, Massachusetts which will be a big part of the story. I'm not a wealthy man but I'm comfortable and I'm wealthy in support from friends and family which you will see during this chronicle. This series of chronicles or essays is intended to be targeted at those who suffered a stroke and those who love them. Specifically, it is targeted at fathers of young children because it is difficult to explain how clear it has become to me about how important they are. My writing style is not for everyone. I will tend to use dark humor, sarcasm, and more than occasional profanity to explain what has happened to me so far. I'm also currently using Dragon software so my flow as not how I usually write. Also, this is not intended to be medical advice or medical chronicle. Obviously there will be a lot of information but to be clear I am not an expert on medical care. This is a personal chronicle intended mostly around the sociological and psychological effects of stroke recovery. It is my personal view and I will only use names of people in positive experiences; for those negative

experiences I'll just identify them by position.
Additionally, I won't let the facts get in the way of a good story; that is, there are not any lies in the story but just my perceptions of what happened – which may not be 100% accurate but above 90%. My friend Brian suggested I use medium.com for this effort so initially this will be a series of blog posts at *https://medium.com/@nyalfuentes*. I welcome any and all comments and questions from friends, family and strangers as I continue this journey of recovery. I'm using the word "I" too much, when really this has become a communal effort. So as we move on, please excuse my pronoun usage.

A little more about me, there are a lot of people whose perfect day would probably be in Paris, the Bahamas, the beach, golf course or any other outing.

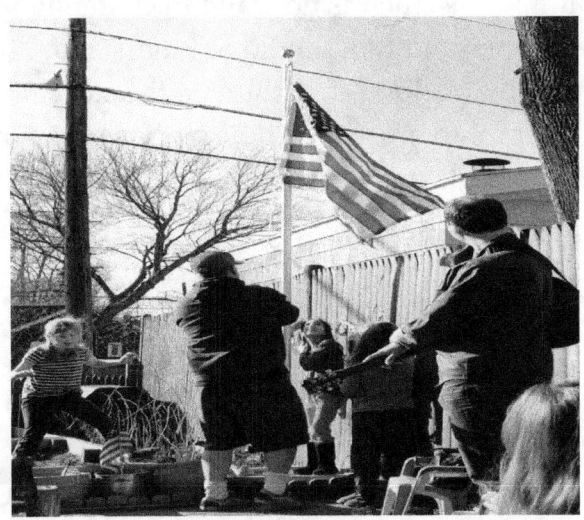

Our flag raising party members Melrose Massachusetts

My ideal day, and this goes to understanding me, is probably to get up early in the morning, fire up my barbecue smoker, go for a 10 to12 mile bike ride, come home, do yard work or other projects, have a bunch of family and friends over for said barbecue, have a few beers, a lot of laughs and good conversation and maybe watch or listen to a sporting event. I'm a somewhat simple person but also desire intellectual stimulation. So that is a little bit of background into me as I begin to tell this tale. Thanks for reading, Nyal Fuentes. If you want to contact me directly, please email me at nyalfuentes@comcast.net

August 2018 Quick Update
As you read through this, realize that most of this was written over a two year period, the combination of past, present and future tense can be somewhat confusing and perhaps even frustrating to those grammarians (of who there are many among my group of friends). Butt too those grammarians, their is no way I'm changing my style. You will see ebbs and flows in hopefulness and hopelessness that help to contribute to the story, I've really made no attempt to grossly edit the story even with better hindsight as to help anyone for whom this may be their miserable albeit hopeful experience.

THUNDERBOLT(STROKEDAY)

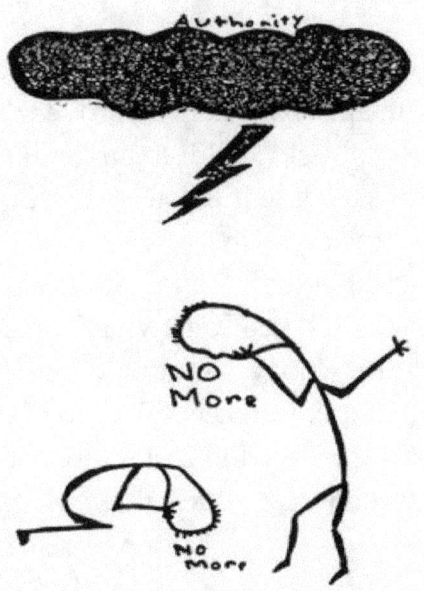

I didn't know it at the time but when I woke up the morning of September 7, 2016, I had the perfect life. I did not live in extreme wealth, didn't drive a Range Rover, live in a mansion, live the life of a real estate tycoon running for president and groping women, but I was pretty wealthy in everything else. I had good health, good healthy kids, a great wife, a good job, a great circle of friends and colleagues, financial security including a home we owned outright, great church, civic engagement, good schools and pretty much had achieved the American dream.

On this morning I was thinking of Jessica Taylor's 20th birthday and my excitement that in one year her dad and I would be able to take her out for a drink and just how much joy I felt watching her grow up. I left the house early to go to Holyoke to visit a couple of schools and confer with the administration.

These trips to Western Massachusetts were not uncommon as we strove as an agency to help improve education for some of our most "at risk" children and adolescents. These are early mornings leaving the house at five or 5:30 to make the most of the day. On the way home I took a conference call and got there in time to have supper with Becky and the kids. Rebecca somewhat ironically went to visit a friend of ours who was getting cancer treatment at Mass General Hospital. I proceeded to go to the basement to lay some flooring for the kid's playroom. The girls played and continued to entertain themselves as I worked.

For some further background I felt completely healthy. I was on no medications, knew I had some elevated blood pressure but continued to try to eat healthy and exercise to control it. As typical with many men of my age I had a tendency -- which I now regret – to not have regular appointments with my physician. Mostly because even though I was somewhat overweight and probably had proclivity to binge drink on occasions, I was generally active always working in the yard, bicycling, playing with the kids and. in a way, I felt I was the healthiest in my life.

I'm calling this entire Chronicle and this chapter THUNDERBOLT because that is the only way I can describe this experience. One day I was a completely functional, active man and then suddenly struck down physically, emotionally, and spiritually. As I will say later in this tome, it has caused both temporary and permanent changes in my actions, feelings and views of the world. Although I've had many experiences that changed my life, I'm wondering if this is the most cataclysmic so far as single time events go

As I was working in the basement, very actively hammering away at tiles and moving heavy objects, I only felt tired due to my long day. Little did I know what was about to come. Suddenly I felt very dizzy and my head felt heavy. I was already on the floor tile. I had no idea what a stroke was and assumed that this was some type of weird vertigo or something. I'd never felt like this before but somehow went up the basement stairs, then upstairs to the bedroom, and removed my contact lenses. As I went to lie in the bed I collapsed to the floor. I grabbed my cell phone and called my wife and told her I was going to dial 911 because something was really wrong and yelled to Elena to grab the landline. She tends to be a little anxious and started to freak out. I tried to calm her down as I called the paramedics.

Meanwhile Rebecca called our neighbor Christy to come watch the kids for a while. Christy is the first in the parade of extremely helpful people in this whole story. The dispatcher asked me a series of questions and shortly after paramedics arrived at my door. I somehow made my way down the stairs and even to the street where I was met by the gurney. When these things happen it seems like every emergency personnel in the city arrives at your front door. The Melrose fire Department and their response was amazing I've come to believe that every cent I pay in property tax is well spent. I was met by professionals competent in their duty and dedicated to getting me to my next stop in the best condition possible. As with many people in the story there's no way I can ever thank them or compensate them for what they've done for me. I felt confident and was joking around about me being a union member and we gotta stick together as brothers and sisters. In a short time, I arrived at Melrose Wakefield Hospital's emergency room.

I was somewhat freaking out. Emergency rooms, by their nature centers of chaos, are the front lines of medical care. Mixed in with people with chronic illnesses, folks who have no other access to medical care, people with serious injuries, folks with medical emergencies like myself and just people who are straight fucking bat shit crazy. It is amazing to me that they can act with the efficiency that they do.

Staff ran me through a series of physical tests which showed that I had very little movement on my left side. They were not positive of the nature of the stroke or its severity and soon hooked up a telemedicine linkup with Mass General hospital. Two neurologists at Mass General ran me through a series of tests, seeing each other through the hook up. They suggested that the pharmacy ready a clot busting drug called TPA. I don't know much about TPA but I've heard it is some kind of miracle drug around clot busting which must be administered in the first four hours after a stroke. Additionally, there is a slight chance of brain bleeding so they do not want to administer it unless it is completely necessary.

At the same time another patient across the curtain arrived in handcuffs and was yelling that his arm hurt and to take the handcuffs off. I empathized with the entire staff having to deal was such nonsense. I suggested to the nurse that I still had one good arm and she should take me over there and I would knock the fucking guy out. Surprisingly she declined.

The next step was transport to Mass General Hospital. As I was prepped for transport, one concern was that I might have of real spike in blood pressure during transport. The EMT and paramedic came into the room. The young man who was the paramedic seemed extremely competent. He asked questions of the nurses and doctors to ensure that he had all the information necessary.

At one point there was a suggestion of a med flight to MGH. I sort of freaked out. Knowing traffic was light at nearly ten o'clock, it would be at most a 15 to 20-minute trip. I did know I didn't want to be med flighted. Who wants their first ride in a helicopter to be strapped to a gurney? Furthermore, they would have to put me in an ambulance anyway because the pickup point was Melrose high school. That just seemed ridiculous to me. Eventually I got in an ambulance and was rushed off to MGH.

Mass General Hospital is an amazing place; the acronym MGH is often meant to stand for Man's Greatest Hospital. Nobody wants to have a stroke but if you're going to have a stroke, have it in Boston. After the marathon bombings, I told my older daughter that Boston is the greatest place in the world. No one who arrived alive at a Boston hospital after the bombings passed away. Our hospitals are known worldwide for the best possible care.

Upon arrival at MGH I was met by probably 20 people – every one of whom knew where they were supposed to be. It was like watching a ballet but without the crappy music. I asked the doctors if I was going to die, and without missing a beat, he said "not tonight." Within 15 minutes, I was brought to imaging where I received an MRI and a CT scan. Reluctantly I accepted the oxygen which they insisted on. Only in these first couple days was I panicked by wires and tubes that were attached to me as necessary parts of the protocol. They confirmed via the imagery that I had a stroke on the right side of my brain. Without going into medical details, generally the right hemisphere of the brain controls the functions of the left side of the body and vice versa; hence my left side paralysis.

The memories of this night and the following couple days are a little hazy to me. I may have to ask others to fill in the gaps. One thing I remember asking the docs in ICU was whether I'd still be able to play the piano. I've been waiting my entire life to ask this "old dad" joke. Without missing a beat, the doc says "well if you are a concert pianist you may lose some of your efficiency but most people get it all back."

Soon after I was put into neuro-ICU to be sure I was medically stable. Rebecca and my brother-in-law Rob joined me in the ICU. By my hazy recollection, probably around 2 a.m., a Fellow from the hospital who was engaged in a study using an MS drug in stroke recovery came into my room. She asked me if I wanted to participate in the study. Being a person who strongly supports science and research as well as my own recovery, I agreed and signed the necessary paperwork with my wife's blessing. Soon I did the initial blood work for that study and was administered either a placebo or the actual drug. It is amazing to me that there is someone on call for a study at 2 a.m. They must really need subjects for the study. This would never happen in educational research.

The first night was such a shock to me that although scared I was nearly devoid of emotion other than some sadness. I am probably what most would call a planner knowing pretty much what I'm doing tomorrow, the next day and the week after that. I have a vague framework in my head of what's happening in five years, 10 years and 20 years, all of which was now being turned upside down. Intellectually I knew this was the best place I could possibly be with the best wife possible leading the way. And so I take the first step of this unexpected journey.

CRITICAL CARE: THE DARK DAYS

These are the darkest days of this chronicle, but thankfully the time I remember least about. I will work on the details as time goes on so please bear in mind this is completely from memory. I was in ICU or maybe it's called Neuro-ICU for a few days and some things remain fuzzy.

At this point I was as terrified as I would be in my whole recovery (at least as far as I know for now). Confined to bed for several days, I had many visits from close friends and family who probably saw me at my most miserable. As a younger man I had probably had bouts with depression and continuing through life some sort of existential depression that many of us have: the classic, why am I here and what is life all about. Generally, though I'm an upbeat, positive person who approaches life with a sense of humor and a seriousness of purpose. I always emphasize the seriousness of purpose. While I may clown around, it is job one to be purposeful and righteous in living my life. In other words, I'm not just here to be a clown. I've developed many strong relationships in and outside of my professional life that are dedicated towards building community and educating children.

Okay that's probably a little bit too much background and I've gotten away from the critical care story. I've never been hospitalized for any period of time in my life until this experience. Hospitals, even as a visitor, tend to freak me out. The smells, the sounds and the general activities create a surreal atmosphere, technology is everywhere and the specter of death and dying is all around. For the first few days I was basically confined to a bed with railings and alarms. At this point my entire left side was paralyzed I could not move my arm at all, my legs, fingers or toes. I had no idea if this was going to be permanent or not, to the point that I cannot even dream or imagine ever walking again. Images of Johnny Got His Gun and, in particular, the Metallica song about it ran through my head. Fortunately, I'll realize much later on that the stroke had very little effect on my cognition or speech. I had and still have slight muscle weakness in my face but that impediment to speech is very slight.

These are the dark days, the days with no hope. Just five weeks later I can look at these days as bouncing off the bottom. If you are reading this as a stroke survivor or family member, at this point in the recovery I can promise you that this is the bottom and it just gets better. You can't see the light at the end of the tunnel yet but at least there is no further train behind you that's going to run you over.

One of the first nights I had a terrible nightmare. I was swimming in a bunch of ropes and wooden blocks. In my dream I cried out to my dear departed Abuela Nieves to take me home. That home being with her in heaven. I tell this story because underneath the tough veneers we put out to the world, we are just one event from crying for our grandmas here or beyond.

The next day during a doctor's visit I related the dream to one of the doctors. Thankfully, I will always have Fred to remind me of what a stupid idea that was. I later learned that for the next two nights I had a 24-hour aide at my door due to suicide ideation. Let me just let you know I'm the last person who would ever commit suicide. I have a love of life and would never consider going in that direction. Nonetheless we have all been hopeless at one time and we just need to look beyond and above for someone to help us.

The desperate always pray and I was among the desperate, I will attempt to cover faith and prayer in a different chapter but the visits from my church pastor Reverend Dominic were extremely important in these early days. As many of us I've struggled with faith my entire life but those early communions of prayer really set a strong foundation for the rest of my healing. Even if you are not a person of religion I strongly suggest communing with someone or some people and have thoughtful reflection to begin healing both physically and emotionally.

At MGH, as in every hospital, there is a constant beeping, people coming for your vital signs and medications and some constant angst amongst all patients. As far as competence. technical expertise and critical care this may be the best place in the world. I do realize how blessed I am to have had this care. One thing about these huge hospitals though is that they are big and there is little personal connection to your treatment or, in fact, what the fuck is going on. Nurses constantly change, individuals come in and out of the room without the patient or family knowing the function of that person.

Occasionally large teams of physicians will come in, a veritable army of doctors in white coats who you eventually identify as the short Asian guy, the Indian dude, the tall blonde babe, the guy with the eyebrows or the really young kid. One never even has the realization of who your doctor is or who oversees your care. I concur with several nurses who advised me to figure out who was actually in charge of my case and the identity of my doctor. In a large teaching hospital there are many residents, medical students, and advanced fellows doing advanced work who are very experienced physicians on the cutting edge. Then there are what they call hospitalists. Hospitalists it may shock you to know are doctors who actually work in hospitals. Additionally, you have specialists: pulmonologists, cardiologists, psychologists and neurologists that will come look at the piece of your body that is yours but that is their specialty. Since then I have learned that the hospitalist helps coordinate all those functions but in your confusion and depression it is difficult to understand that.

Like me, few know what a stroke is or feels like before it happens. One thing about a stroke is that there is no physical pain involved. Most physical pain comes from a fall or accident caused by the stroke. One thing I learned in this first couple days was to listen to your nurse. To be honest at MGH, the only real connection I made to hospital personnel was the nurses. Nurses are a unique combination of angels, highly skilled technical professionals and your mommy when you are scared of the dark. It is an incredible amount of love. Throughout this chronicle of experience, I would be neglectful to not think of the nursing profession at every corner.

The one incident that was painful physically came two or three days into my stay at MGH. I was transferred to the restroom and onto the toilet as I executed a bowel movement. The nurse instructed me on two things. First, do not lean forward. Second, do not wipe your butt. Having done these things for over 40 years I did both and the nurse's left arm could not stop 230 pounds of fat ass Puerto Rican hitting the floor headfirst.

In an instant about 12 hospital personnel crowded the restroom picking me up off the floor back into a wheelchair. Apparently, the venial sin of the hospital is a patient falling. I think if I had had a .45 caliber pistol and shot up the place there would've been less of a response. This fall caused an enormous black eye with an egg above the left eye nearly shutting it closed. This added insult, ugliness and pain to the injury I already suffered. It would be the only physical pain I would suffer during this whole ordeal. In fact, the only pain medicine I received at any hospital was a small dose of Tylenol for the eye. Essentially for the next few weeks this nearly shuttered eye would drag along with my already half withered body as a telltale sign of stupidity. It looked awful. I'm not sure how anyone looked at my face. However, it served as a lesson for the rest of my hospitalization: always listen to your nurses!

Hygiene and Humiliation

Not meant to be gross or scatological, this information on bodily functions may be one of the most important topics for many. For instance, how much we take them for granted. For the past 40+ years I've generally been capable of using the restroom by myself, showering by myself and taking care of the day-to-day responsibilities of being clean and presentable to the public. If you are friends and family of a stroke patient or any patient hospitalized is important to realize a few things.

Toilets can be deadly. You don't realize how much of a gift being able to have a bowel movement, wipe your own ass, wash your hands and walk out of the restroom really is until you are unable to do it. The ability to get out of bed walk into a bathroom and pee standing up for us gentlemen is something we just assume will always be there.

As I said previously I had a toilet fall in my early days at MGH. This fall, along with injuring myself, made me very reluctant to use the toilet again. For urinating they give you a plastic bottle constructed for that purpose. Eventually you learn how to pee in it in bed without dripping/spraying urine on yourself. I've always hated the smell of urine. As I often tell my wife, it just smells like poverty. It smells like Park Street station, it smells like Central Square on a hot summer day and generally is just depressing. One of the worst situations at this time was getting up in the morning and having just those few drops of urine on your pants. This raises the issue of how taking a shower is about as easy as the invasion of Sicily. Eventually you master this skill but always live in fear of knocking over the bottle reaching for eyeglasses, the remote, what have you.

While in rehab I lost all my appetite for a week and a half and, to be polite, I couldn't poop. Both things were completely new to me, I was like a clock both eating and excreting. At Spaulding the quest for me to have a bowel movement became a team-wide goal for my nurses. Every hour or hour and a half they would come in suggesting that I use the toilet. Early on just using the toilet, just getting there, took an enormous effort. I had to be dragged up to my feet, placed in a wheelchair, pushed into the bathroom, and basically female handled onto the pot. Again, I was warned, don't lean forward, don't wipe your own ass.

For several days nothing happened, they began to give me Colace and eventually Jill made me a prune juice and milk of magnesia cocktail. I've made some strange drinks in my life, but this took the cake.

Nurses are obsessed with bodily functions. If falling is the ultimate sin in a hospital, not moving your bowels or urinating regularly is just secondary to that. My nurse Jeannie was in on the deal as well. Jeannie is Filipina and one of the friendliest and nicest persons I've ever met in my life. She was always smiling and no matter how disgusting something might be, she would be whistling show tunes and singing songs. She had Sesame Street scrubs and would say things like "don't worry honey it's a natural process." After threats of further intervention, including a suppository, I eventually took care of business without leaning forward or wiping my own butt. With the same smile on her face she would give her own children, she cleaned me up and got me back into bed. It is important to remember that while for the patient these are entirely new experiences, for nursing staff it's just routine and they want you to do it as they ask.

As I started to have some mobility, they would leave me alone in the restroom. It was extremely liberating being able to wipe my own butt and pee standing up. I still needed an escort to the bathroom but could do it on my own. This all sounds pretty gross and somewhat graphic but this humiliating process is a very difficult part of the recovery that is overlooked and important to understand.

Showering was a complicated process as well. Whereas a teenaged boy might think being assisted in the shower by good-looking women is alluring, in fact, it just adds to the humiliation. Early on it is nearly impossible to get dressed and undressed without a lot of assistance. You really don't realize how hard it is to take off your pants with one arm and another leg that won't function well. Five weeks later I'm still showering in a chair at my home but I am able to get out of the tub fairly easily and wash myself, dry myself and get dressed.

At the rehab it was nearly impossible. The first few times I took sponge baths and tried to avoid daily showers which are ordinarily the only way I am allowed to get out of bed. Again, staff at the hospital are used to this; it's nothing out of the ordinary to them. Clean up someone and move on to the next guy. Luckily, with one good arm I was able to brush my teeth, shave, wash my hands and other daily dignities. Others don't even have that. Showers are important though, as they loosen your muscles for your daily therapies and are refreshing. So another word of advice: when offered a shower say yes.

A major part of Occupational Therapy, activities of daily living, I referred to as adventures in daily living because they seemed so impossible at the time. Heed your OT's advice wisely and you'll be on that toilet in no time

When your spouse or other loved ones are given permission to assist, let them assist. Again it is going to be uncomfortable and humiliating, but you love them, they love you and you want them to help. I imagine for us dads that have seen our wives go through childbirth we may have one up on the rest of y'all.

In conclusion, dealing with bodily functions is going to be humiliating. It is going to suck, and other than the physical disability, it sucked the most about being in the hospital.

NOT THAT KIND OF REHAB

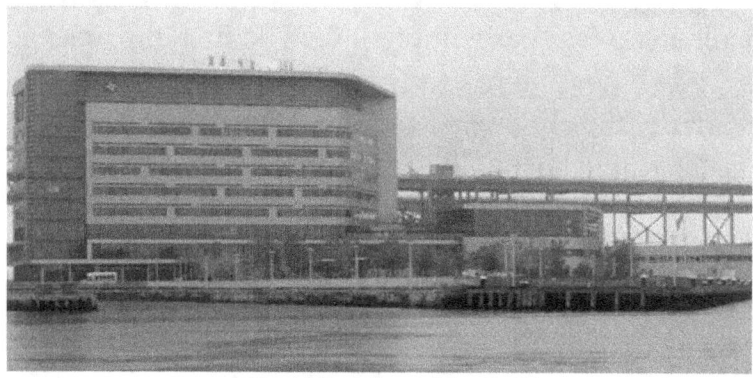

Spaulding from Mystic River

If you knew me as a younger man and someone said I was going to rehab, you would've probably anticipated someplace sponsored by a former First Lady or a short stay at Gosnold on the upper Cape.

On Sept 11th I was medically cleared for transfer to a rehabilitation hospital which I took to mean you're a cripple but you aren't going to get more crippled. I took a much less professional ambulance ride from MGH to Spaulding rehab hospital in Charlestown. These guys bitched for 45 minutes about their job, their coworkers, and their bosses which is exactly what you want to hear barreling thru Boston helpless on a gurney. At this point my entire left side was essentially still paralyzed causing me to be dumped from the gurney into another bed like an enormous bag of rice.

Rehab has a different feel to it. Most people don't have Ivs. The incessant beeping, other than assholes trying to get out of bed when they are not supposed to, is gone. Parades of platoons of doctors coming to see you treating you like an exhibit at the Topsfield fair do not really exist. No more constant awakenings for vitals. If a hospital can be so, Spaulding is more comfortable and you start to be treated more like a human being than some smart kid's science project. I have a single room with an incredible view of the Mystic River and Boston Harbor. The room even has a minifridge. And a bathroom. This was the hospital that Mayor Menino went to and in his name there is a beautiful playground outside the hospital in Mayor Thomas Menino Park.

On the wall there's a whiteboard that says all the stuff you can and can't do physically along with the primary people involved in your care. Having a couch for your visitors makes it seem like one of those long-term motels, just without the kitchenette.

People start to introduce themselves and for the first time you can identify your doc. There is humanity at the core here, not just extreme technical competence. First, they do an evaluation to get a baseline. My report was probably that I can lay in one place like 200plus pounds of crap and shout expletives in two languages and cry like a lil bitch. Now I understand that establishing this baseline is critical for the therapists to determine my course of treatment.

Spaulding is world renowned. It is where Saudi princes fly to for their rehabilitation. There are many different floors in Spaulding. My particular floor was dedicated to strokes and other stroke-like symptoms. Other floors are for spinal and cervical injuries, comprehensive injuries such as multiple amputees, a pediatric floor and floors for people with things like hip or knee replacements. I was lucky to be placed in Spaulding. Generally, people stay here for three to five weeks and then either go to a skilled nursing facility (nursing home) or are sent directly home. The median age of my floor was definitely over 70, although there was a 23-year-old man from East Boston who had a minor stroke and a couple folks in their 30s or 40s who had been admitted. Many of the nurses said the stroke floor is the best environment because people actually got better, not always the case for some of the other floors.

It is difficult to express how much Spaulding Rehabilitation Hospital is responsible for helping me turn a major corner.

First, I met Dr. Lee who appeared to be the coach of the many people involved in my care. He always had this little sheet of paper in his pocket. He knew everything about my care, knew everyone I was seeing and had a basic plan moving forward. At all times I knew who was in charge and it wasn't in that godlike way that some physicians have. He knew his spot, like any good coach, and each team member had to actually execute the plays he designed. It was rare to see this combination of bedside manner and technical expertise in a doctor – confidence without the arrogance. He told me the average stay was 17 days and then hilariously explained to me, the data analyst, what an average is, that some stays were longer and some stays were shorter. I think in this instance I would've probably gone with the mode.

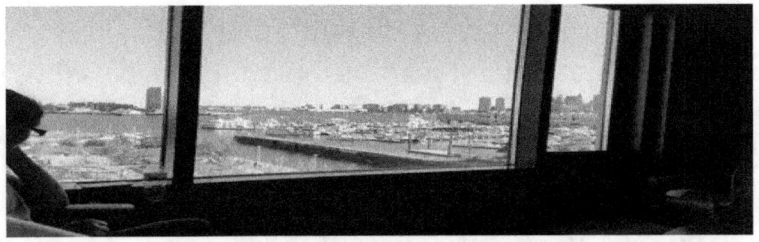
I never really appreciated this view
as much as my visitors did.

The nurse's names are written up on the board, although we have substitute nurses from time to time. Due to scheduling, I have three to four nurses that always seem to be there. Most of these women were very young it seemed to me. Well, I mean for nurses – wasn't like a bunch of Elena's running around the hospital. My love for my nurses is not easily matched. To deliver medicines, to explain things to you and tuck you in at night. I will never be able to thank people like Christina, Jeannie and Jill enough. They will continue to play a part as this journey goes on.

Whereas other rehabs may vary, my experiences pertain to Spaulding. Nurse's aides are critical to the recovery process. They help you get showered, use the bathroom, get dressed, get your meals and everything else you can think about. Most of my aides were wonderful. At one point there was this older woman from Peru named Rosa, who reminded me of my grandmother in a loving and pious way. She prayed for me at Padre Pio's heart and encouraged me to eat in the way that only a Hispanic grandmother can. Eat, you need to get strong, you need eggs and toast, not fruit and yogurt. Okay, so they are not cardiologists.

I would urge you to be observant with some staff. One or two per diem aides did not read the board that details the patient's strengths and weaknesses. For example, one aide didn't seem to know that I could not walk and had no strength in my left side. She was asking if I could just walk to the bathroom. Because I had no cognitive issues, I understood what was going on with me and could monitor my own care to some degree. However, many people with strokes have cognitive issues and can't be responsible for overseeing their care. Be sure you and your loved ones can trust your entire team. If you note someone not checking the board or knowing your capabilities, you and your loved one should report the infraction to the appropriate supervisor. Not just for myself, but I did it out of concern for my fellow patients.

In a perfect situation you'll be assigned one-on-one therapists for Occupational Therapy, physical therapy and speech and language. In addition, you will likely be assigned to several groups -- a stroke support group, Occupational Therapy groups, patient education and perhaps a speech language group. Additionally, Spaulding has what is called a recreational therapist which is more along the lines of things that are fun but involve rehabilitation, more on that in a later chapter.

A basic introduction to therapies. For strokies, physical therapy is mostly about mobility. If therapy can be fun, I found physical therapy the most engaging. Since my right arm was very functional I learned that you can do a lot with one arm. You can't do a lot with one leg despite my daughter's insistence that I could hop around.

Occupational Therapy or Erika's torture is about getting your arm back to normal. If you have not lost function in your arm, you never realize how amazing your arm is and how much complicated movement it can do. I was also involved with speech and language therapy. Luckily, other than some muscle weakness on my left cheek, my speech and cognition were unaffected. Nonetheless the cognition exercises in preparation for the neuropsychology exam proved very helpful and complex thought is believed to help rewire your elastic brain.

A week after my stroke and two days after entering Spaulding Hospital my night nurse Jill was giving me my nightly meds and daily pep talk. Jill is one of these classic New England girls, smart, blessedly rough around the edges, sarcastic, funny, and pretty. The kind of no-nonsense girl you wish your friends would get together with. Though she is relatively new to the profession, becoming a nurse just a few months ago, she seemed to have the knowledge, skills and heart of a much more experienced nurse. We bonded quickly. That Wednesday the 14th I moved the toes on my left foot. I asked Jill, "am I moving my left toes." She responded "yes." I replied" fuck yeah." Then she said "Fuck yeah. Can you imagine what you can do next week?"

So, this was my introduction to Spaulding and turning the first corner.

STARTING THE HEALING: THERAPY GODDESSES

Once medically stable and at the rehab center, the next step is to start to come back. Rehab, or come back, I would best describe as combination of medicine, rest, a positive attitude and lots of work with your therapists.

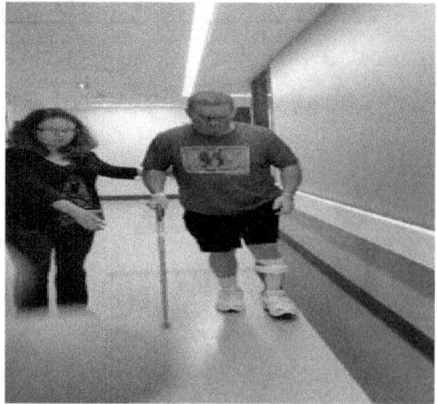

Although I've touched on it before I do want to give a brief description of each of the therapies as I see them.

Generally, there are three types of therapies for stroke patients, depending on your particular weaknesses. The first is physical therapy, which is basically the work you do to get your mobility back. It focuses on the legs which as you know have dozens of different muscles and tons of nerve endings that really work together to help you walk or, as the joke became, ambulate. Ambulation focuses on a few different things: strength, control, flexibility and what I found to be the hardest so far, balance. As with everything here, you don't know what you got till you lose it.

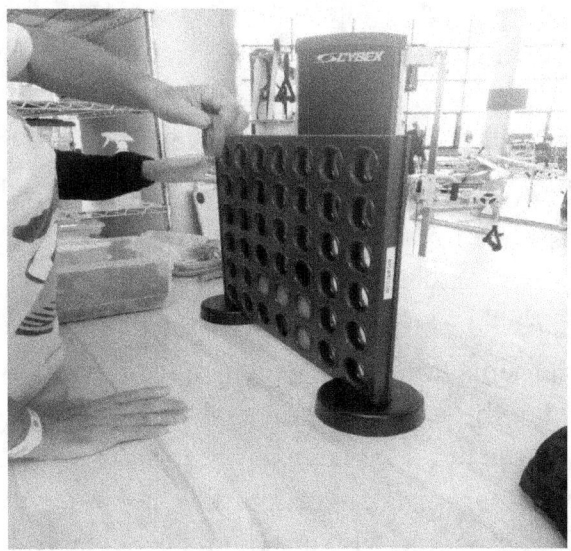

Occupational Therapy, or torture as I like to call it, has to do with strengthening the arms and functions of daily living. Again, the arm is an incredible thing. Look at your arm and think about all the motions it can do. If you're reading this concurrent to your stroke and lost one side, use your good arm and note how you can move your fingers, thumb, and wrists in all directions including rotation, moving your elbow back and forth and nearly full rotation of your shoulder. In daily life all these things work together to be a functioning human being.

Speech and language for some may be the toughest and only concern from the stroke, depending on where the stroke was located in your brain. Fortunately, I have very little disability around speech, language and cognition. As I met others, I realized that my physical disability was easier to bear than those who had speech and cognition issues.

Three young women -- my therapy goddesses – helped me along my journey. Again, to Molly, my physical therapist, Erika, my occupational therapist and Hannah, my speech and language therapist, there is no way I could ever compensate or thank you for starting me on my path to wellness.

At the beginning of the stay there is the evaluation to see what movements you can do and what you can't do in all aspects of the three different areas. It will be mostly a repeat of all the other stroke examinations you've had so far but these therapists are different. They are truly healers, taking people who are medically cleared to start down that road to renewed health. They are your personal coaches, your mentors of movement, pep talkers, and support for everything you will need for the rest your life. It is somewhat frustrating at the beginning because there's a good chance you can't really do anything. It may start out with you lying in a bed, trying to move your fingers or foot and slowly being coaxed out of that bed which you may think you will never leave. It's that frustrating at the beginning, a few weeks ago I never imagined that I would ever even stand up again, much less walk or operate as a normal human being.

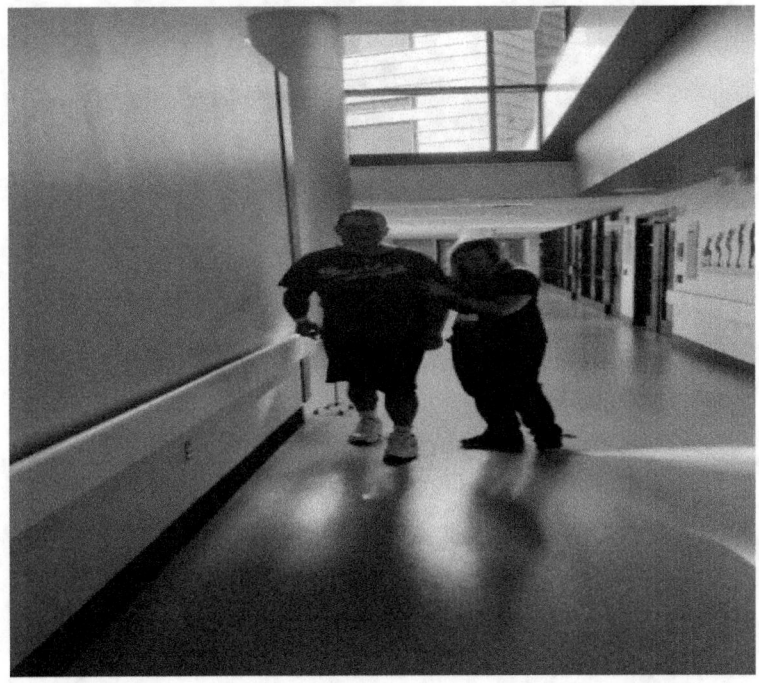

It is an incremental process and continues to be for me. Improvements are so small you may not even notice them, which is one reason to have a therapist taking notes. It may be some additional strength in your ankle, being able to touch a finger to the thumb, brushing your teeth, grabbing your phone with your bad hand or something else very minor like that.

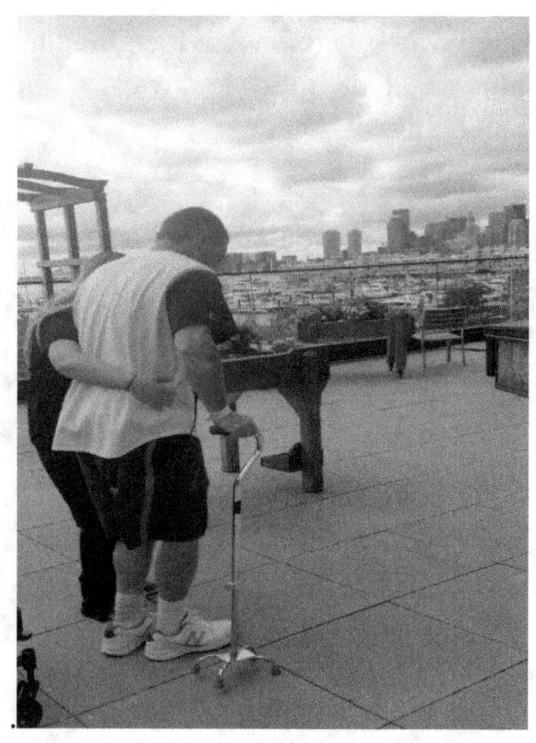

First I want to talk a little about Molly, my physical therapist, and what she did for me. I told this directly to her face when I left the hospital: she saved my life. She took me back from the abyss, put me on my feet and taught me to walk again. Now I may not run the Chicago Marathon juggling the entire way, but four weeks after the stroke I managed to walk into my six-year-old's birthday party on my own albeit with a cane which was my first goal.

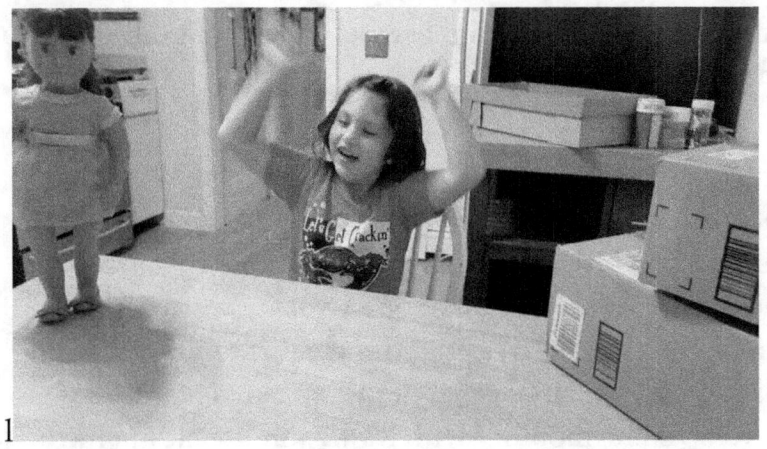

1

Molly is in her mid to late 20s, blonde, pretty and with a
smile that lights up a room. She is dedicated to her craft,
caring and is a true healer. Part of this job is psychological.
You need to make sure that people are confident that they
can do it. Part of it is being a salesperson. You need to sell
the fact that each one of these steps leads to a greater thing;
that eventually you will be back on your feet and assume
normal activities. This is a hard sell – particularly for
people who have been really active prior to the stroke. You
just can't imagine ever getting back to where you were.

I met with the PT person, usually Molly almost every day
except for Sunday. Sundays are a day of rest at Spaulding.
Molly would take me down to what is called the
gymnasium. The gymnasium had room to walk, many
machines and served all the patients at Spaulding. It was a
busy place. You would see tons of patients from other
floors and really start to realize how good you have it. You
would see young, very fit men who were paraplegics, folks
who were multiple amputees and people whose roads
were much longer than mine for even the most basic of life

functions. You would almost feel a sense of guilt that you had so much.

Physical therapy consists of a lot of exercise to strengthen the muscles in the legs and improve balance. Every day things got a little better. She would let me ride the recumbent stationary bike for a while to warm up, hold the bars for balance exercises and then eventually let me start walking with a large cane. Pretty quickly I started to develop some mobility with Molly kinda holding me up, leading to my starting to walk with a cane. It was one of the most liberating things I ever did in my life. For all intents and purposes, I was free. Molly was right there beside me but just had a hand on my back. She trained me to climb stairs, keep my head up, eventually move to a single cane and even ambulate without it.

Mostly it was about continuing to increase my confidence and at least see the light at the end of the tunnel. We would joke around a lot and she got to understand my personality which was super helpful because some people would think I'm kind of a jerk in that I can't shut up and I'm constantly joking around. It is hard work though. You really have to be thoughtful of every movement, every heel strike, every bend of your knee as you move forward. At first it fucking sucks, then slowly you become inspired. When asked if I needed a break I always said no. I told her to" push, push, push." She was much more patient than I was. Eventually I started to walk pretty well with a cane, but it really is exhausting even today for even the shortest walks.

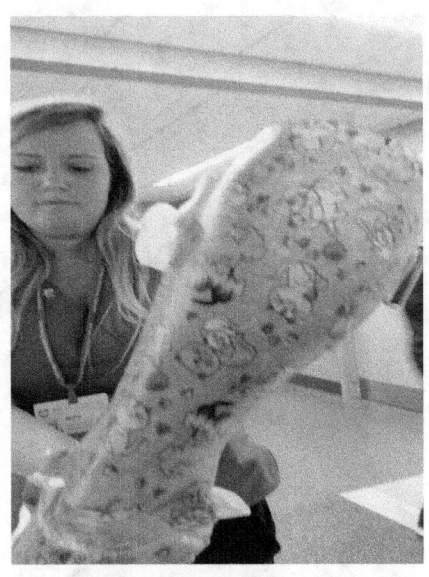

A couple weeks into my stay, Molly noted that a brace might be helpful to keep my ankle from dropping. One of the hardest parts about learning how to re-walk is not dragging your foot along the ground. Spaulding has a brace shop on the first floor where I was custom fitted for a brace to keep my foot from dragging while still allowing the ankle to strengthen. Since you were allowed to choose a design for your brace, obviously I wanted the most ridiculous one possible, so I chose cats. The brace specialist said I was the first adult to ever get the cat brace. One thing I learned in the struggle is not to take yourself too seriously and that humor no matter how black is necessary for survival and recovery. If offered the brace, take that opportunity. I only wore it for a few weeks. While it was very helpful in general walking and gait training, I found it to be difficult climbing stairs and other activities that need more fine controls of your ankle and leg.

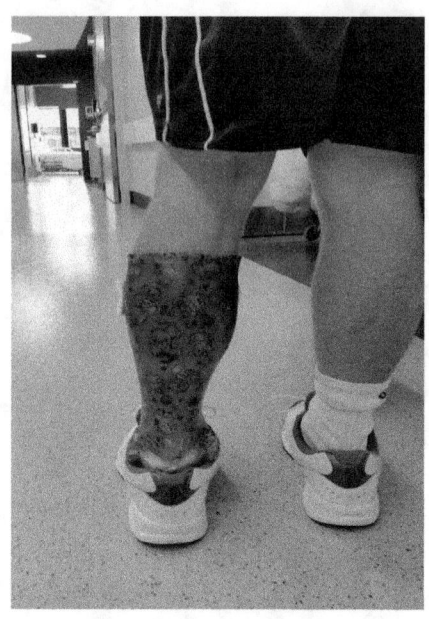

Occupational Therapy, I found to be torturous. At first, I had very little grasp, strength or control to my arm. Much of occupational therapy has to do with playing children's games. We would play connect four, use peg boards and clothespins and in the height of all evil, try to pick sticks up off the table. Erika was my occupational therapist; this young lady should never have to hear the cursing that I used ever again. I let her know I was cursing at myself, admonishing myself and trying to get the stupid arm working. Try to use your weak arm in everything you do.

Another part of Occupational Therapy was getting back to daily living. Learning to shower, get dressed, use the restroom and things of that nature. I'm certain that somewhere in Occupational Therapy school there is a torture clinic, and that Erika could easily be hired by the CIA or foreign government secret police to extract any information she wanted. It's really that difficult. The growth is much more nuanced than mobility, mostly because you can do everything right handed if you have a left-hand weakness. There are a lot of exercises for strength, flexibility and control but to be honest it involves a lot of children's games, so if you have kids, playing Shopkins, Legos or any other games will become part of your OT once you return home.

With Erika I sometimes felt like a bad patient. As much as I liked her and knew I had to do it, I dreaded OT every day. Even now five weeks later I'm dreading the arrival of my OT later this morning. It's just that difficult albeit essential. At one point, while I was taking a shower, I reached for my deodorant. Erika moved it further away. To her every little thing was an exercise in getting me better. She helped me learn to get in and out of a regular bathtub (there is a mock apartment located at Spaulding to practice), get dressed and in another pinnacle of torture, relearn how to tie my shoes.

In addition to the one-on-one Occupational Therapy, there is something called OT group. This is less focused on specific OT skills and more about socialization, memory and some type of activity. For the most part I would be among the youngest people here, which is a big part of the story anyway. We play name games, do the daily news, and then usually have some type of silly thing going on like playing hockey on the table, corn hole, or some other activity involving dexterity and attention.

The last piece of daily therapies involved speech and language. As I've explained, I had very few deficits in speech, language, and cognition. I met with Hannah who evaluated me with several standardized tests. She also reassessed me around swallowing. Passing the swallowing test is critical as it allows you to eat whatever you want within reason. Gradually she realized I didn't really have any serious deficits. She assigned me some cheek and mouth exercises to strengthen the muscles in my face that have been affected, but mostly worked on cognition. There are tons of memory exercises, stories and the like. I tried to tell her I can't even do these exercises sober.

Speech and language does assist with general brain function and helping with the elasticity of the brain during your holistic stroke recovery as the brain begins to rewire itself. I would read speeches and she would record them into a host of cognition exercises. Some of them again included games at one point to test my divided attention. I was listening to a podcast while playing snap circuits. Afterwards when I assembled the circuit, she asked me questions about what happened in the podcast. Much of this is to determine if you're okay to return to work. At one point I received work materials from our agency website about ewis and educational proficiency plans. After a short time, I was dismissed from speech and language therapy and assigned to other therapies that I was weaker in.

So these are the wonders and struggles of daily therapies. My advice: eat well, work hard, have a strong positive attitude and develop a good relationship with your therapist. Furthermore, don't lie to them. They are your best friends right now

Day by Day: an extended stay

"So you're gonna be institutionalized
You'll come out brainwashed with bloodshot eyes
You won't have any say
They'll brainwash you until you see their way."
Suicidal Tendencies

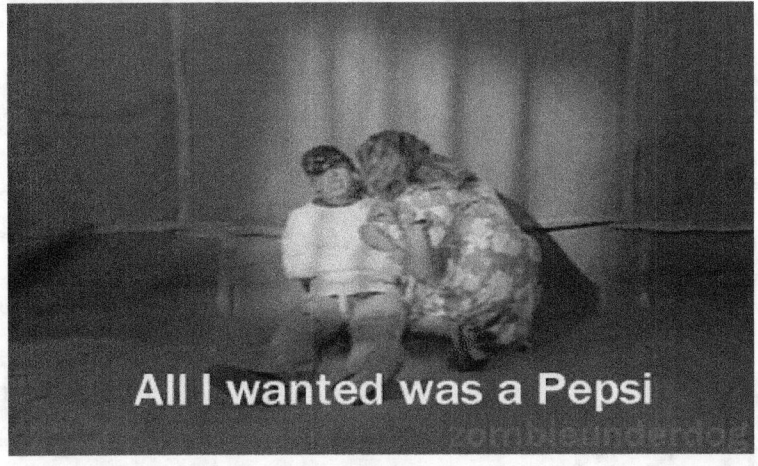

All I wanted was a Pepsi

In my life, I have spent very little time as a patient in the hospital. A car accident here, food poisoning there. I spent a couple nights when my kids were born, sitting in an uncomfortable chair next to my wife plotting escape, but other than that, I've been pretty lucky.

Between the two hospitals, both MGH and Spaulding rehab, I ended up spending 27 days in the hospital. Twenty-seven days, almost an entire month. I could have never imagined being in one place, or in this case two places, for so long. It's not like being imprisoned. People are nice to you, generally treat you with respect and don't necessarily blame you for being there. However, there is a sense of confinement. You don't really know for certain how long you'll be there, even when they set a release date. Just the sense of having a release date makes you want to start writing on the walls.

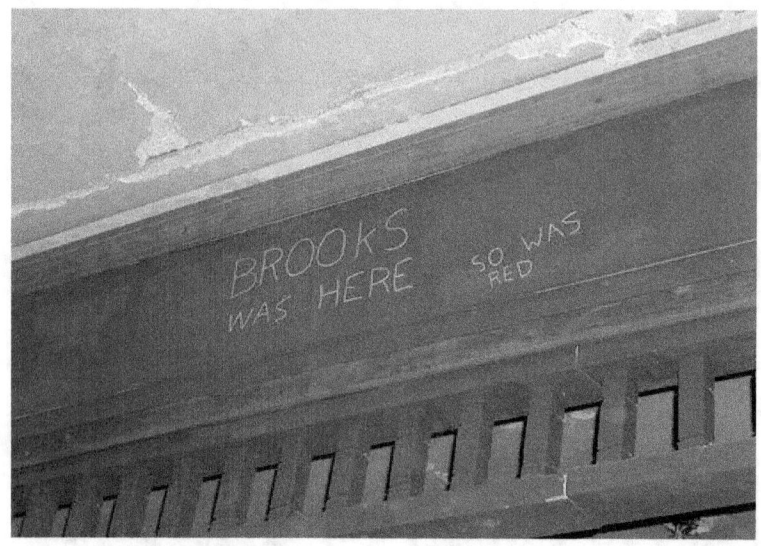

Most of this essay will concern Spaulding Hospital, the time I spent at MGH was short but to be honest pretty traumatic, if in fact you can define a posttraumatic event as trauma. As I said before MGH was about getting me medically stable, patching me up so that I could start healing. Basically, just making sure I did not get worse. Also, it was the darkest time, I was just really not sure what the hell was going on. My stroke was on a Wednesday; by Friday they began to wait for a spot at Spaulding to open so I could transfer. The aforementioned fall off the toilet and black eye were among the low points of these days. The fall was entirely my fault and I then learned to listen but my anxiety for the next step in my journey increased. Generally, it is difficult to get a space in the rehab on a weekend, staff is smaller, and it is more difficult to open a space. On Sunday, they told me I was getting transferred on Monday. I think it was the first time that I had any sense of optimism. Monday morning, I was transferred by ambulance to minimum-security, I mean Spaulding rehab.

Generally, it is difficult to get into the rehab facility on a weekend. Staff is smaller and it is more difficult to open a space. On Sunday, they told me I was getting transferred on Monday. I think it was the first time that I had any sense of optimism. Monday morning, I was transferred by ambulance to minimum-security, I mean Spaulding rehab.

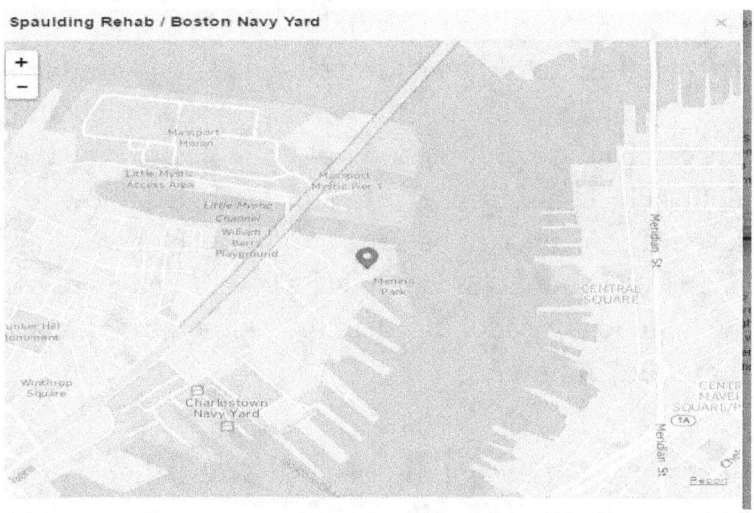

Spaulding, as I've mentioned before, had much more humanity to it, to the point that you are actually greeted at the front desk while being wheeled in on a gurney. The first thing most people noticed was the view of the Mystic River and Boston Harbor. I still felt like an object just being dumped from bed to bed. Slowly, my attitude began to change a bit, I realized that although this is a long journey, I turned a small corner.

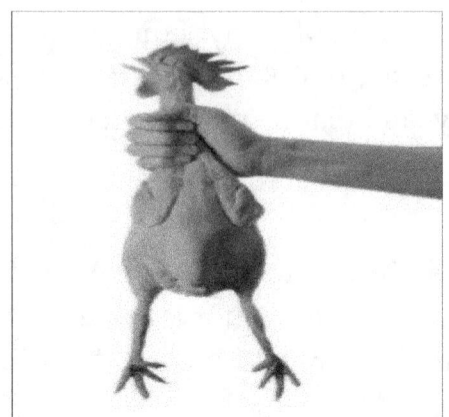

Now you really start to think of the basic essentials of life, like eating. For the first 10 days, I didn't have much of an appetite, which if you know me is a pretty strange concept. Looking back, I wish I had brought some hot sauce. Most stroke patients are put on a low salt diet. I don't tend to eat a lot of salt anyway but institutional food is pretty bland. The vegetables are pretty good but I'm not sure how they made the chicken so rubbery. In fact, I googled "how to make chicken rubbery," because in a lifetime of cooking professionally and at home I never did it. If you want to know, you do it by cooking at a high temperature for a long amount of time.

When eating, like everything else in a stroke, there is always a degree of difficulty. Eating in bed is not as fun as you might think. Dropping food on your clothes just becomes an embarrassing fact as time goes on. Because I passed the swallowing test, I could pretty much eat whatever I wanted albeit if it was from the hospital menu it was going to be low-salt and generally low-fat, with pretty damn small portions. Initially all I was really eating was small fruit cups and a little juice. It's all I could really handle. There was no real physiological reason and no diagnosis, I just really had no desire to eat.

That first Friday evening, even though I had no appetite, my friend Matt brought me pulled pork eggrolls from a bar called Ironsides and even though there was no appetite they were just too damn good not to eat. I would soon discover that food from outside is going to be essential, cardiac diet be damned. None of the nurses had an issue with bringing outside food. Generally, they knew that happiness and strength were so important in recovery that the occasional culinary foolishness fit into the entire program. Plus, if you had extra, staff seemed to always appreciate the offer of food, even if they didn't take you up on it.

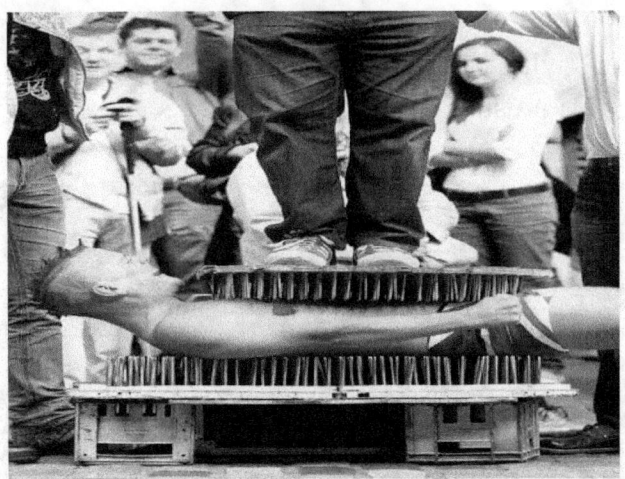

Sleeping in a hospital sucks. I don't ordinarily sleep well anyway but I got very little sleep in the hospital. At first I probably spent 90% of my time in bed. I would recommend getting out of bed as soon as possible even though you will basically live in a wheelchair for a while.

Becky brought me two nice pillows from home as I tend to be a pillow hoarder.

Because you can't move very well, you will probably be tucked in at night usually after nightly meds. There were some points in the hospital that I was going to bed at 7:30 after switching on the Sox. There's just a lot of things you can't do so you may as well go to sleep. The problem became even though I was taking trazodone for sleep, I would sometimes get up very early in the morning like 2:30 or 3:00 and not be able to get back to sleep, basically tossing and turning until normal morning came. One night I woke up at 10:30 PM thinking it was time to get up. Even though I had a window and beautiful view of sunrises and sunsets it really didn't matter to me; time of day was irrelevant unless I had a therapy appointment. Not to go all Foucault on you, but there is a certain life philosophy that comes with incarceration even when it is meant in your best interest.

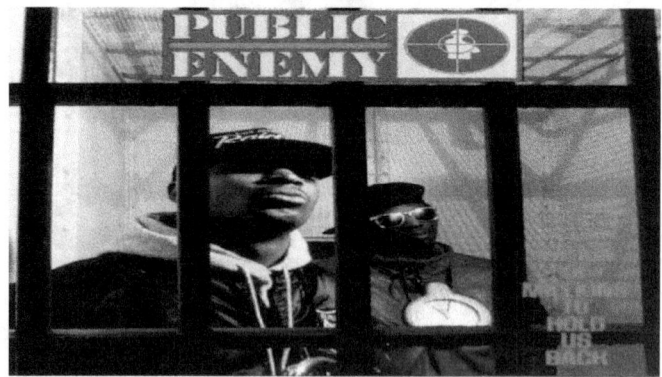

To be clear, hospitalization is not prison. There is no intentional punitive factor to it. Even at Spaulding, with a great deal of personalization and love, odd things happen.

Things that just wouldn't happen in the outside world. For example, there was this one woman I called the ass lady, she appeared to be the woman at the hospital that was in charge of bedsores. (I can't remember the technical name.) Somewhat irregularly, I don't know her schedule, she would come and check your body for sores. She noticed a small abrasion at the top of my butt crack and instructed me in care for said butt crack. I told her not to worry and thought that I may have come in with that. She was the only one in the hospital who actually seemed to yell at me for something. I fear the ass lady's visits in the same way you would fear a high school assistant principal. You knew you were in trouble for something.

Outside of being in bed you likely will spend much of your day in a wheelchair as it is the easiest way to get you around from therapy to therapy, to the restroom and if you're just hanging out. Being in a wheelchair isn't super comfortable. You always feel like you're in transition, kind of like sitting on a bus. It's not terrible but you know you're on to something else later and the dude next to you is looking at porn on his phone. Not really but work with me here. You are usually whisked from appointment to appointment by the therapists or by aides. You sit here while you eat lunch or supper or just hanging out. I chose not to watch any TV other than sports. Daytime TV is a desert. I have a particular hate for Wheel of Fortune. The man next to me played Wheel of Fortune on a very high volume and I literally felt sick to my stomach.

Mostly I communicated to the world through Facebook, reddit, twitter, and other social media. During my down time, I texted and listened to an occasional podcast.

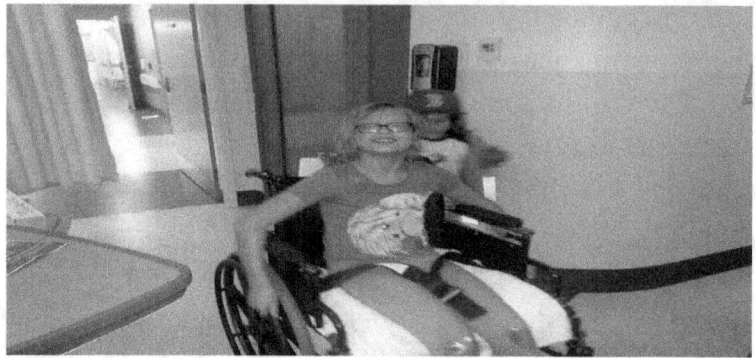

Visits are crucial, particularly from my children, as I was feeling pretty shitty as a dad. I treasured every person who came to visit me and was extremely blessed with many visitors from family, friends, colleagues, my church family and others who spent their time driving up and paying to park to spend a little time with me. If you are a friend or family of a stroke patient keep the visits up. Honestly sometimes I was so tired I wasn't really a good host and at about 7:00 p.m. I would start to fade. I can't say enough about all my visitors – those that brought me meals, gifts, but mostly those that brought me joy. My colleagues from work would keep me up-to-date on the day-to-day events and ensure me that my work was being taken care of which was very important to me.

Intellectual stimulation is an important part of stroke recovery. As a visitor it is a bad idea to talk to a patient like they are child. For those of us with physical weakness, our minds are still sharp even if our reaction may be a little slower than usual, mostly due to being tired. For younger patients such as myself, much of our social interactions not with staff are with people that are considerably older than us. We look forward to our visits with peers and normal conversations about the outside world, particularly when we are sharing meals. Eating alone sometimes makes you feel like a loser.

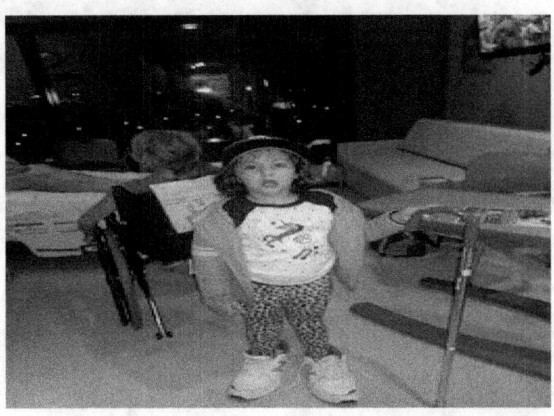

A few days after I went in the hospital, I started to break the world of the institution into two groups: crips and norms. Crips were my people, people who had suffered strokes and had visible disabilities to them. Norms could be a lot of different people. Certainly, it was staff but mostly it was visitors, outsiders. [Early on before I realized the idea of cognitive disabilities and stroke, people who could just amble into a meeting without assistance.] In some cases, it was difficult to ascertain if people were crips or norms, but I have to admit I was jealous of the norms, people could just get up go about their business without any restriction. I think to this day I still harbor some jealousy as I watch other parents at the soccer game jog, and jump around as they watch the children.

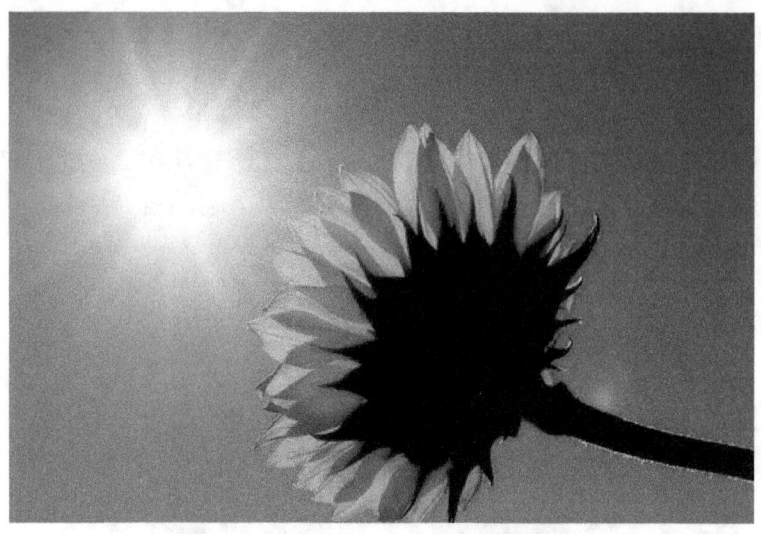

During your stay, a positive attitude is most essential. Several patients were angry, even spiteful and you knew their road was a lot longer than yours. I spent most of my time in groups joking, flirting with the old ladies and chumming around with the older guys. Why the fuck not, you got a choice in this. You can be a miserable bastard or you can move towards that light at the end of the tunnel.

THE LIGHT AHEAD OR YOU GOT THIS: THE POWER OF POSITIVE THINKING

"Everything can be taken from a man but one thing: the last of the human freedoms — to choose one's attitude in any given set of circumstances, to choose one's own way." — Viktor E. Frankl, Man's Search for Meaning

As an adult, the secular books that have shaped most of my life philosophies include Viktor Frankl's *Man's Search*

For Meaning and George Orwell's *1984*. Both these books were written from a sense of desperation. Frankl's rises above terrible situations and documents amazing stories of overcoming them. Orwell's piece, although fiction, illustrates another man attempting unsuccessfully to combat his desperation. In no way am I comparing my situation to the survival of a concentration camp, but often we need extremes that help to identify the norm.

For those that haven't read *Man's Search For Meaning*, Frankl was a psychiatrist who survived the concentration camps and later documented the experience by pointing out what people had done to help others while in the camp. He documented the humanity in the worst of situations, i.e. a man giving his last handful of bread, so another could survive.

While I cannot quote this book chapter and verse, the imagery resonates in my head every day – that is the ability of any person to choose his own attitude in any situation. We see this every day amongst our daily heroes, whether they be teachers, police, parents, soldiers or anyone else operating in what sometimes can be a very chaotic world. In my experience as a counselor in urban schools I would often define this to students in a different way -- a more controllable way. I would tell them" learn the game, master the game and then change the game," particularly when faced with the challenges of classism and institutional racism. But I digress. All of us have periods where we are down, we feel oppressed or that someone or something is against us. I attempted to stay positive, sometimes successfully and sometimes unsuccessfully.

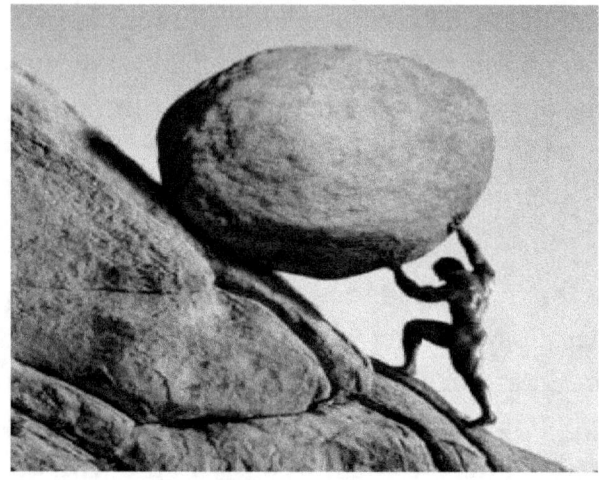

My strategy as a more adjusted adult than young person has mostly been to maintain this positivity with frequent but truncated bouts of negativity and stress. I used Facebook as a kind of journal during my stay in the hospital. Sometimes my general positivity in life is due to having a very strong foundation, a strong wife, relatively happy family, great friends and a good job. I know this isn't all accidental. I worked hard, got an education and managed all of my strong relationships while attempting to get rid of most of the negativity around me. We joined a progressive church based on love and support and we attempted to ignore all that would bring us down. This doesn't happen every day; some days really suck.

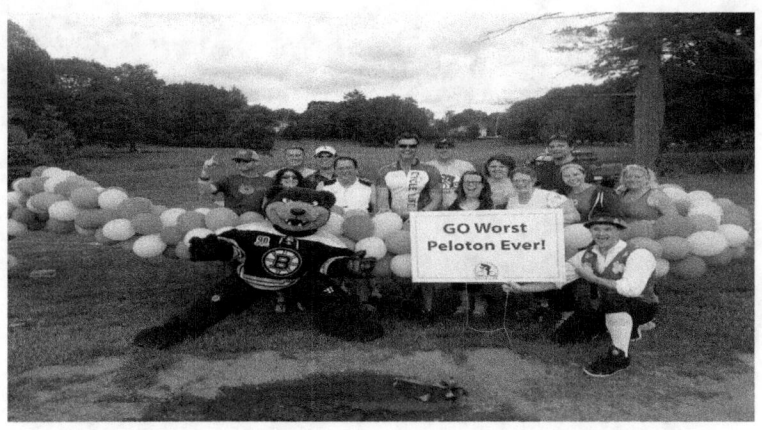

This foundation for even the ability to be positive in the hospital was built thanks to many others. During my health episode I was grateful to my union and the labor movement in general. Because I was able to bank my sick time for 15 years and have great health insurance. I could concentrate on getting better and not losing everything I've worked for in my life. I know others don't have that privilege

There is a mythology in this country of the rugged individualist. By most accounts, people would probably consider me to be bright, hardworking, pretty strong and "tough" physically and emotionally but this can happen to any of us. I am blessed to have this soft-landing into a safety net. Regressives want to tear this safety net apart. Vote wisely people and think of those who don't have it as "easy" as I do. As they say in Scripture, for whom much is given much is expected. A small part of my effort to give back is the construction of this blog.

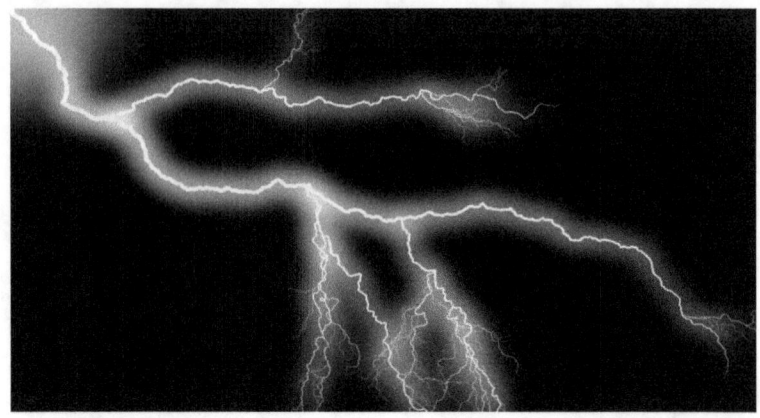

Back to the matter at hand, when this first happens, it is impossible to be positive. It is the thunderbolt, the burying avalanche, the tornado that metaphorically knocks you to the ground. I think for many of faith, the first thing you say is "Why me, God?, I'm your servant, why did you knock me down when I'm truly trying to do your will." Atheists will often bring that up as well, if there is a God why did this happen?

Strokes have nothing to do with God; they are a quirk of human physiology. What happens afterwards, the universal oversoul of those around you, of those who support you is where God is. At the beginning as I said earlier, there are prayers of desperation which soon turn to prayers for strength. Early on, I texted my friend Terrell and asked for the prayers he used during basic training. He sent them and I used them as part of my initial recovery. But this is not a religious tract, for those who are now tuning out, it is just part of the story.

The initial days of a stroke are fucking terrible, there's just no way to say otherwise. You are buried in a hole in the darkness, desperate, with no way out. Any attempt at positivity seems ludicrous. You're completely defeated emotionally, spiritually and intellectually. After a few days you don't yet see the light at the end of the tunnel but you see the tracks below you and realize no trains are behind you. This is really important, because until you get to rehab you likely will be in this state. Once I got to rehab I began to see stroke victims that were way worse off than I was, but also those who have moved forward. The nurses, doctors and therapists talked about what the next few weeks would entail and that people with strokes got better. Soon I made the decision -- I was going to not only become a stroke survivor but a stroke defeater. I was going to kick this motherfucker's ass.

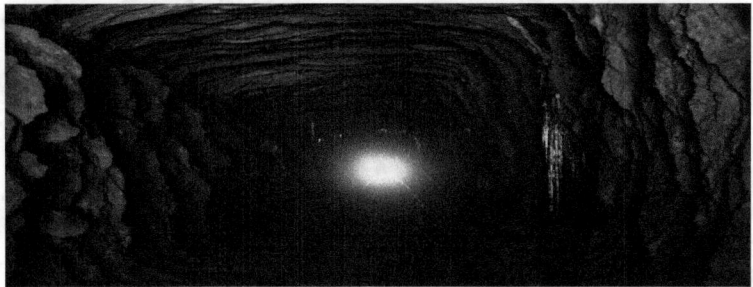

These are easy words to say to yourself in your head lying there not being able to move your arm or leg and a whole other thing to maintain it for a long period of time. The psychologist said many stroke survivors suffer from severe depression after about two months. So I gotta keep an eye on that but for now my outlook continues to be positive and I am moving forward.

.

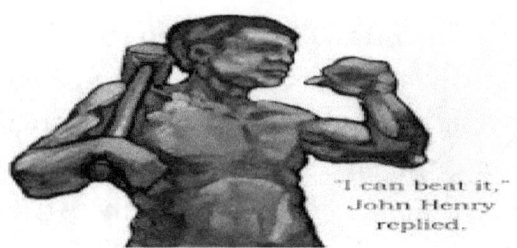

"I can beat it,"
John Henry
replied.

I'm not pretending to be some type of tough guy. There were many times that I would cry, often at night when I was alone or in the morning when I woke up. Sometimes when kids left or talking on the phone to my mom I would well up or just cry for no reason. Being positive does not mean not bowing to that crazy emotion of sadness from time to time. It's more of a general attitude and not a 24/7 thing.

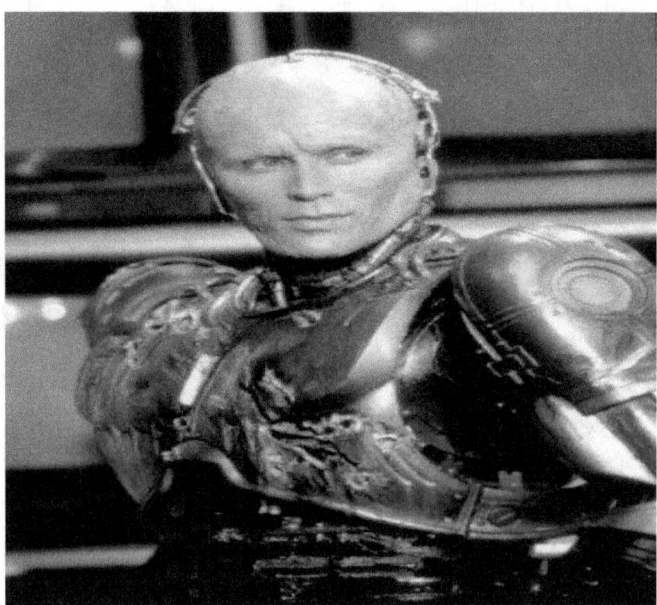

One morning in my twisted mind I spent a considerable amount of time between pining for my kids like a little bitch and obsessing over the movie Robocop in my head. The brain works in strange ways. Fighting depression is not a game, that motherfucker wants to knock you the hell out. I did not find the psychologist to be super helpful but your experience may vary. You can always ask for further help.

In groups you would see many people who had sort of given up, so I tried to clown a little bit -- do stuff like talk about my kids to try to bring up the morale in these groups. There are many people, particularly the older white guys, who really seem to have just surrendered or thought that the miracle of modern medicine would save them. Any medical professional in the hospital – doctor, nurse, aide, or therapist – will tell you will tell you that a strong, positive attitude is necessary for healing. Stroke recovery has a lot to do with the work you put in. By not being a cranky douche bag, you will find that your therapists work even harder with you, that your nurses pay you more positive attention and that your aides are more helpful. It's human nature to help those who are easier to help and willing to help themselves.

I also really have to thank my Fuentes hardheadedness and stubbornness during the beginning of this journey and its rare usage in good instead of evil. This positivity is not a firework but a slow burning fire within you. No matter what you need to do to keep up your spirits, do it. For me, talking shit with my boys, hanging with my girls, posting to Facebook, eating good outside food with friends and family all helped to keep me going. But mostly it is going to be the fire inside you that keeps you moving forward -- the willingness and strength to get you back to normal, however you define that normal, and live a great life ahead.

Ambulation

We walked around the lake
And woke up in the rain
And everyone turned over
Troubled in their dreams again

Visiting time is over
And so we walk away
And both play dead then cry out loud
Why we always cry this way?
The Cure

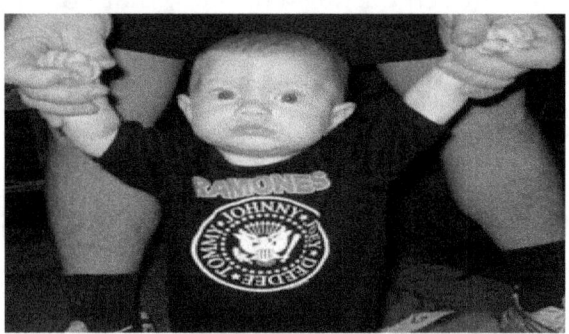
Elena learning to walk

In many ways this is just an addendum or extension of my conversation regarding physical therapy. There's a little twist here because this is really dedicated to one of the earliest functions of human evolution – bipedal transport. Walking on your own two feet is really underrated! There are tons of things you don't realize, among them: peeing standing up, being able to go short distances for daily function and ultimately being able to use walking as a form of transportation.

When I was at Spaulding, I thought about the many times that Elena and I and sometimes others had made the walk around Charlestown to the USS Constitution and later on to the north end for lunch. These are some of my favorite days. Elena loves the Constitution Museum and the vessel itself and has a particular love for a couple stops in the north end for Italian food and gelato. Thinking about doing these walks again seemed very distant. Early on in my stay I was a "maximum assist pivot" – that is with my one good leg and one good arm I would be hauled up onto that one leg turned around and dropped into my wheelchair. As long as I can help it, I have no intent to ever be a wheelchair again. Granted it was my rickshaw to the world and after the first couple weeks in bed it really felt good to sit up and be rolled around, but I spent a lot of time in that chair. Being whisked off to therapies and to meetings and the occasional trip outside it really made you want to get up and walk.

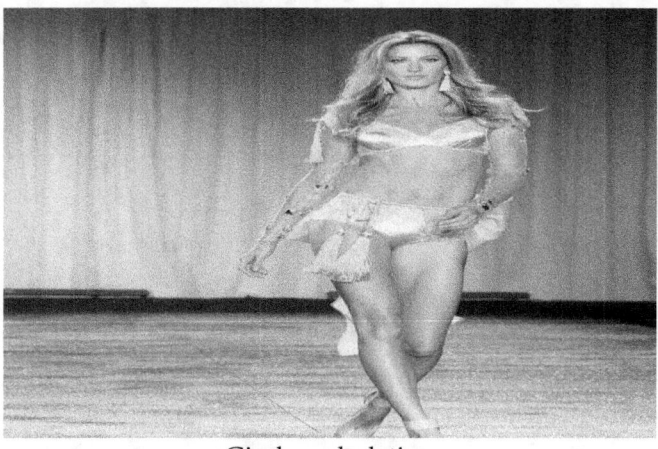

Gisele ambulating

In the past 10 years, I have helped both of my children including the one above to learn to crawl, walk and eventually run. As I recovered, I realized how difficult it is to learn to walk. Now I know how tired and frustrated my kids were and how they wanted to go back to crawling. And imagine doing it with a leg that is completely frozen. Early on when I was in bed being the somewhat dirty old man I am, I suggested to my friend Christie that if Gisele Bundchen was five steps away from me and told me to grab her boob I would still fall straight on my face. Then again, even under the best circumstances, that might be true. I know about "sexist pig" and "too much information" but sometimes that's just how I roll.

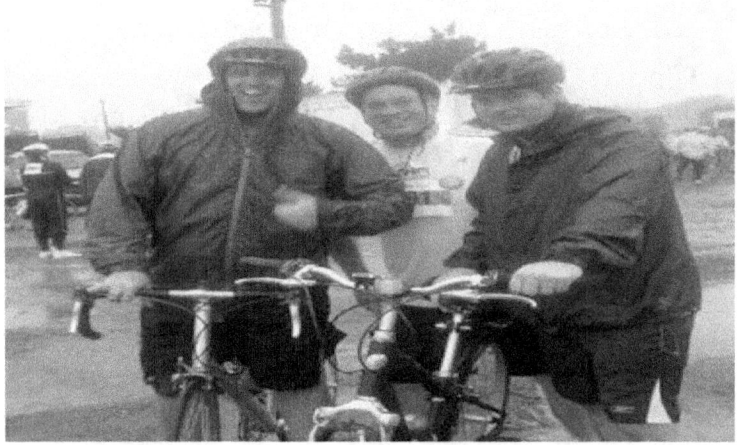

Soon after I was describing this to my occupational therapist in another way. Saying to her that me walking across the room right now would be the equivalent of my good friend Fred Ebbett doing a Simone Biles floor routine down the hallway. She doesn't know Fred but the giggle I got was enough to give me strength for the rest of the day. For context Fred is the tall guy in the left of this photo so if you don't know him you probably can imagine this super tall, as my mom would say, oversized friend tumbling across the floor.

"Max assist" as referred to above basically means you have nothing, you can't do crap. And it's put up on the board to politely tell other staff that you really are a worthless piece of shit when it comes to any type of movement. My goal initially was a get them to change this board. To the best of my recollection, you soon graduate to minimum assist pivot and then close contact (a therapist holding it up as you walk), close guard (walking beside you in case you lose your balance) and that is with or without cane to eventually work yourself up to the ultimate which is independence. They eventually also cleared my wife to be close assist and this gave her the pleasure of occasionally escorting me to the restroom.

As I stated in the therapy chapter, Molly was really responsible for getting me going, well that and just having the persistence to keep moving. On my right arm, I have tattooed the words *siempre palante,* which essentially means "always keep moving forward" in Spanish. Or in the English language vernacular, "keep on keeping on." These words are on my arm as a constant reminder to not sweat anything and keep on going. My ancestors were pounded by weather, war, colonialism, hard work in the cane and coffee fields, yet always kept going until my life was possible. Recovering from something as cataclysmic but relatively minor compared to those circumstances should be a cinch with the resources I have.

Enough of the soapbox, walking to me became job one. I became obsessed with it. I could not wait to see Molly in the morning and do the various exercises we had to. I usually insisted on three things during the sessions: keep pushing me, I'm not going to say I'm tired; let me have a little shot at the recumbent stationary bike so I feel like I'm alive, and let me at least try to walk either with a cane or holding the bars.

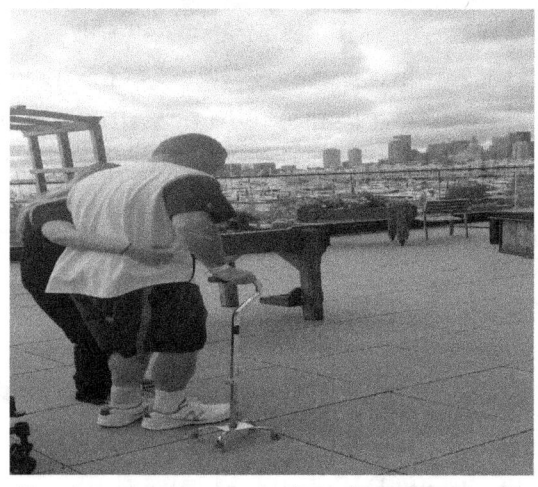

On September 21, just two weeks after the stroke I turned a corner. That day I took some steps outside without physical support in PT, with Molly there to coach and catch me in case. I told people that was the day I started to feel human and the subject rather than object of the sentence. As Churchill said after the second battle of El Alamein -- not the end or even the beginning of the end but it is the end of the beginning. I was feeling all positive thoughts and prayers, a light around me as I did it, those few steps in some ways were a sort of punctuated equilibrium to set my walking evolution moving forward quickly. One of the exercises was a timed very short walk probably less than 10 feet that included getting up out of the chair walking the distance going around the cone and getting back in the chair. The first time I did it with the cane it took me about a minute and a half. Yes, a minute and a half is what it takes for some sprinters to run about 600 m, but I was probably going six. The next week however I did it in 32 seconds and later 27 seconds which still is ridiculously slow, but improvement. Incremental improvement is really what it's all about. You have these huge pieces like being able to stand up from a chair and from then on it is as Marisol would say "slow and steady wins the race." Visitors coming was one of the rare times that I would break the rules. On occasion when a visitor walked in I would show off by standing up out of the chair and giving them a hug or if appropriate a kiss. I imagine if the nurses saw this it would annoy them but it was one of my few transgressions while in the hospital. It was super important to me to give back a little bit of the love that had been given me and to maybe give some of my visitors a little hope that all the support had helped the payoff.

Eventually in the gym I started walking a little bit without the cane and then one day I walked about 150 feet without a cane. I was using a smaller, one-pronged cane at this point, my balance was getting much better and I got more confident each day. They really want you to walk with the cane because one of the most important things is to redevelop your gait. I had a pretty screwed up gait to begin with. My mother has a similar gait and it is all about walking on the balls of our feet instead of going heel to toe like normal humans. While this is probably great for sports like basketball and football, it's really terrible when you're trying to relearn how to walk. Essentially not only trying to remember how to walk, but also trying to unlearn the mechanics that I had for more than 40 years. This is still a struggle for me. It just feels weird even though I can probably walk about 40 minutes with a cane some six or seven weeks later.

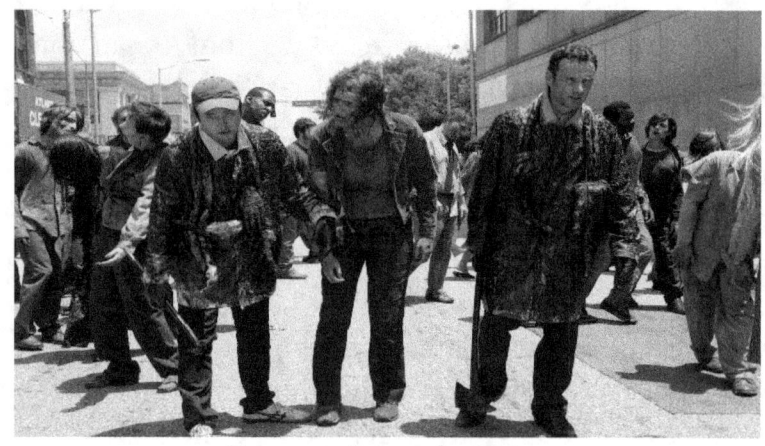

Community ambulation

Soon Molly started talk about something called community ambulation. Community ambulation is the speed at which normal people would travel. From someone who tends to walk a lot, commuting from place to place, shopping or just everyday business running from meeting to meeting, I tended to walk at a fairly brisk pace. The goal for community ambulation was about 1.9 mph which boggled me as it was like standing still. It got worse though. Molly put me on a treadmill set for .9 mph. In other words, it would take me 66 minutes to walk a mile. Still it was just practice and all practice is good. She would set up small obstacle courses to work on side-to-side mobility and assure that I was looking from side-to-side and up, and not just watching my feet. It's funny what actually becomes an obstacle. It was really a struggle just to step over a 1-inch dowel on the ground or to take my clown-sized feet **around** some small cones.

Eventually you advance to the community ambulation level and I mean you're really cooking. You realize the easiest part of walking is actually your normal strides. The challenges come with walking around things with small steps and moving side to side. Also moving in confined areas, not to mention steps and stairs, is challenging. These are the things that you also don't realize when one step seems like climbing Mount Monadnock, and the steps you use to get around the restroom or in the kitchen come back gradually.

Restoring this takes a lot of work holding the bar and practicing sidestepping and assorted exercises to really work on your balance. For me strength came back first, making it fairly easy to ride the recumbent stationary bicycle or get out of the chair. Balance and control were two different things. At some point, my left foot seemed to be insubordinate to my wishes. I would physically try to send a message from my brain to the leg. Even to this day I think about every step, still sending a message from my brain to my left foot to land where and how it is supposed to. It's very strange when it just seemed like a reflex to make something such a thoughtful process.

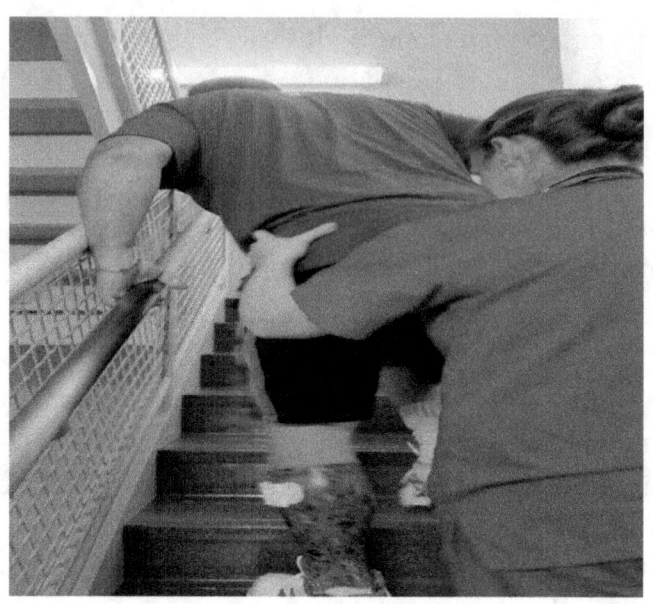

I did get the opportunity while at rehab to walk on different surfaces: grass, pavement, inclined sidewalks and ramps, inside and outside, all of which took different efforts to master. Among the most challenging were stairs. Stairs were an integral part of the training and exercises. Rehab has these practice stairs with strong railings on each side. At first each step seems unconquerable. The therapist is right beside you ensuring you do not fall. Eventually my left leg was very strong, not much weaker than my right leg albeit with terrible balance and control. The first thing you learn is good leg to heaven. This means your strong foot should always be the first up the stairs and the last one going down the stairs. One therapist told me "you are gonna fall, so learn how to fall right. Never fall down the stairs. You can fall up the stairs as it won't be that far, but if you fall down you are back in the hospital."

I was at somewhat of an advantage by being young so that a simple fall on grass or even on a carpet or wood floor would not be extremely debilitating. For older people or people with brittle bones this may not be the case. I've fallen a lot in my life: doing stupid shit, wrestling, tripping over stuff, falling off my bike after getting hit by a car, slipping on ice all the way down my front stairs with recycling in my hands and done all right. I learned how to fall: cover your head, break your fall with one of your extremities and roll into it. So I had something going for me.

But one word of advice: mind the stairs – it is where true disasters can happen. I practiced on the real stairs at Spaulding and got stronger and stronger. I was lucky enough that my friend Nick installed both grab bars and a beautiful railing going upstairs at my home. It may not be karma. It may be the beer and barbecue that ended up paying off in the struggle.

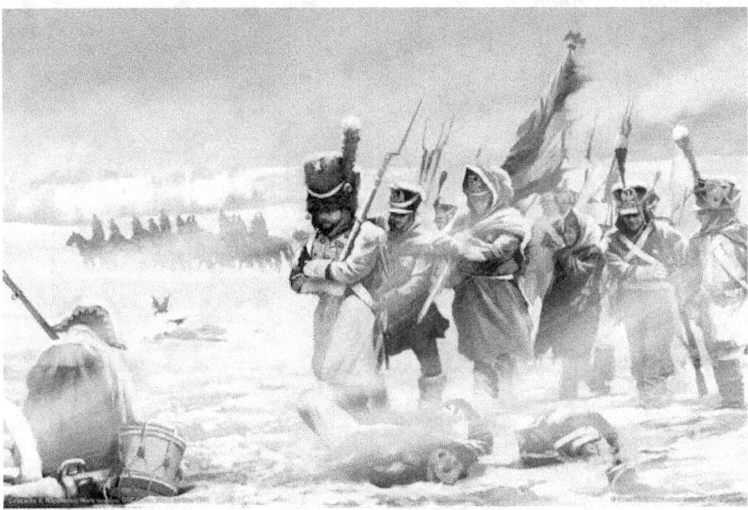

Learning to walk again in a proficient manner is very important to me. I realize it will be a struggle. At some points I feel like some of Napoleon's Imperial guard marching back to Russia through the cold snows, feet going into puddles and somehow miraculously sinking into some mud that is yet to be frozen despite the cold Ukrainian winter. But you will make it home, to rise again and serve Napoleon or not.

FRIENDS AND FAMILY: WHAT DID I DO TO DESERVE THIS REDUX

One child grows up to be
Somebody that just loves to learn
And another child grows up to be
Somebody you'd just love to burn

Mom loves the both of them
You see, it's in the blood
Both kids are good to mom
Blood's thicker than the mud
Sly and the family Stone

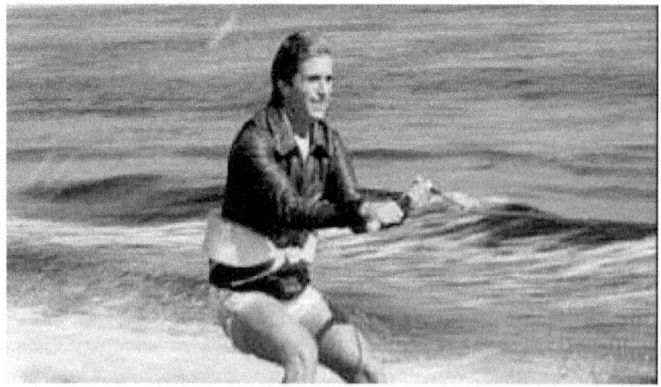

As I keep writing, I fear this is going to turn out like many efforts at media end up -- you run out of steam and all of a sudden you are out of plot lines. The next thing you know Fonzie is on water skis in California trying to jump the proverbial shark. [This entry may be one of the most important for me to write and I feel like I'm going to screw it up.]

Most the time when you say, "what did I do to deserve this?" it has to do with something really shitty that happens to you. You look to the sky or out over the horizon and look for what invisible enemy has set you back. In my case, it is entirely opposite. I'm not quite sure how all these pieces fell into place to give me such a strong support system of friends and family. I'm worried about writing this piece mostly because as I name names other people might seem forgotten so let me start with a holistic thank you to everyone. All of my friends, family, church family, and colleagues near and far did more for me as a collective than any of you can imagine.

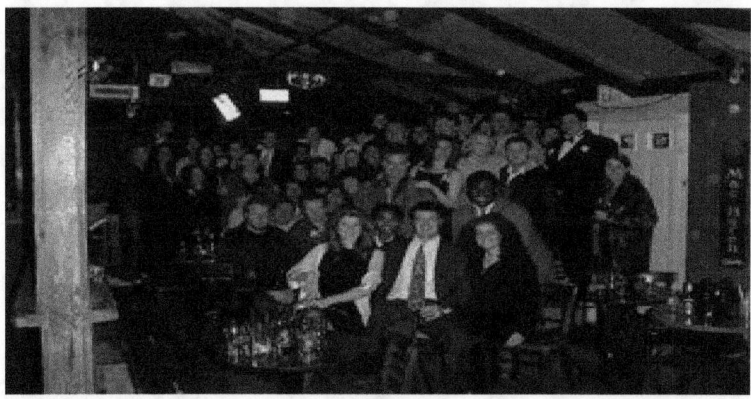

wedding

So to reprint something that I said in the moment on Facebook, I want to first express my gratitude to my friends and family, every visit, Facebook post, note on a card, message, and text has been critical towards my attitude, morale and healing. The help around the house with my usual chores, care for our kids, the prepping for me to come home, keeping my work stuff going, the food, well it is impossible to state how humbling it is. Work friends, Lincoln friends, Melrose friends, family from far and near, Umass peeps, neighbors, my Cameron crew, friends I've had for most of my life, worst peloton ever, my church family. I can't name them all and probably would have another stroke from exhaustion trying to thank everyone individually. If Rebecca Fuentes has been my rudder and anchor, y'all have been in the bottom of that trireme guiding me through probably the darkest seas of my life. Also to the people all over the east coast, people I haven't even met of all faiths and creeds praying and thinking of me. I as a person who struggles with faith have felt your light and it has strengthened me.

This whole situation sucks but out of it I have learned that I am truly loved and have managed to build strong lifelong relationships that I value more than you can ever believe. Again thank you for everything. I will never be able to repay this debt.

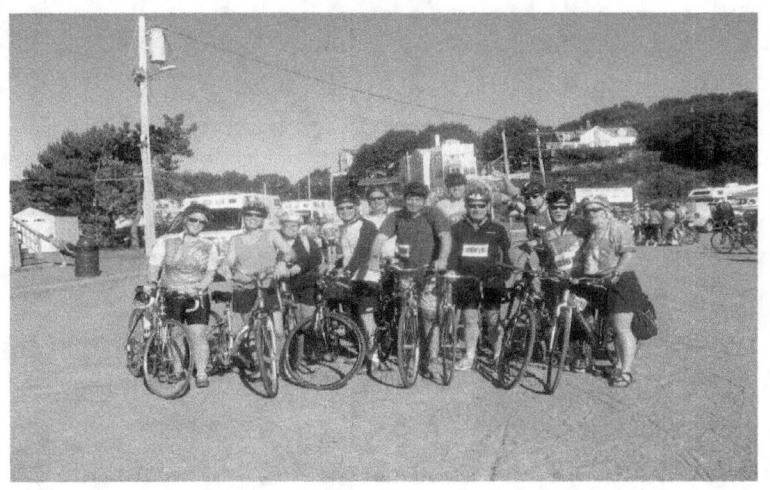

I don't think I can write it any better than that. I mean I could fix the shitty syntax and grammar in there but that really came from the heart and in the moment, plus visualizing y'all in the bottom of that boat rowing to hard-core punk music really kinda makes me laugh.

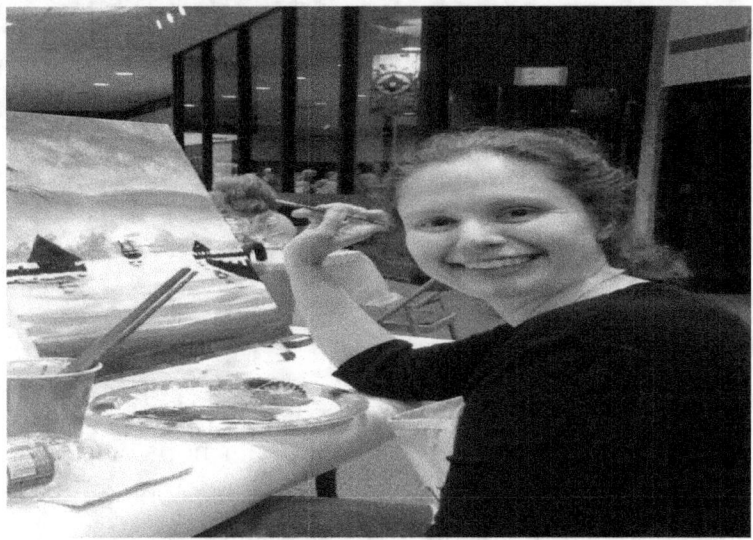

dedicated public servant and fine artist to boot

I could never say enough about my wife Becky. She managed all of our affairs, handed me tissues when I was crying, reassured me, and did everything imaginable to make me feel loved and cared for at all times. A lot of time in the hospital, you just feel like a useless piece of shit and that you will never be normal again. She was there at every opportune time to shovel me off the sidewalk and help keep me relatively whole. She helped me to see that light at the tunnel's end and showed that she, me and the girls were headed to that light, love and our perfect life together. On my best days, and these certainly were not, I can be kind of a jerk. These days were much harder and she kept it altogether. She was Princess Leia to my C-3PO.

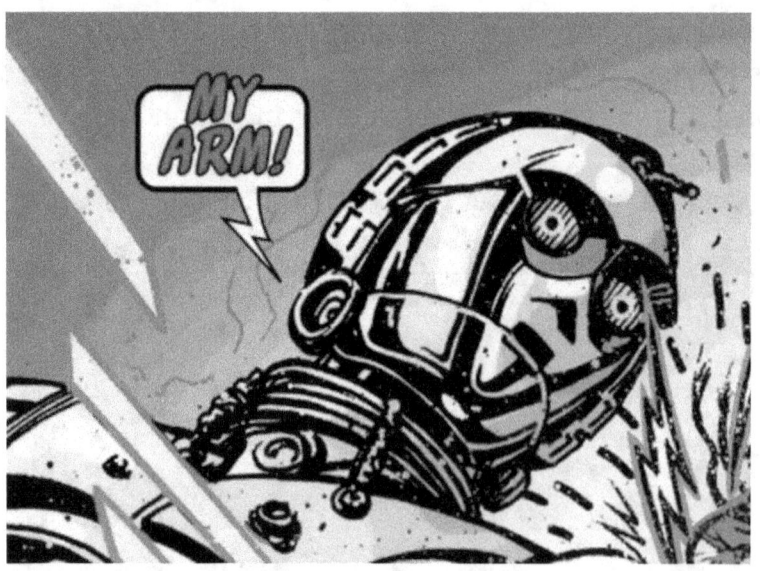

Early visitors when I was in MGH saw me at my worst. During the time I was there I had an enormous black eye which quickly spread to my other eye. I was one ugly fuck. People kept visiting, bringing food, joy and positive conversation. For other stroke victims, their friends and family; one thing visitors need to remember is that the days of a stroke patient are pretty busy. We soon tend to "fade" as time goes on. It is not a reflection of the company and we want you to stay. In fact, the more conversations that are complex and involve using your brain help in the recovery as my system retires itself so you don't need to talk to the person like they are my six-year-old daughter Marisol. I for one still wish I had the energy to thank all my visitors individually in my usual verbose manner but I have treasured every one of them.

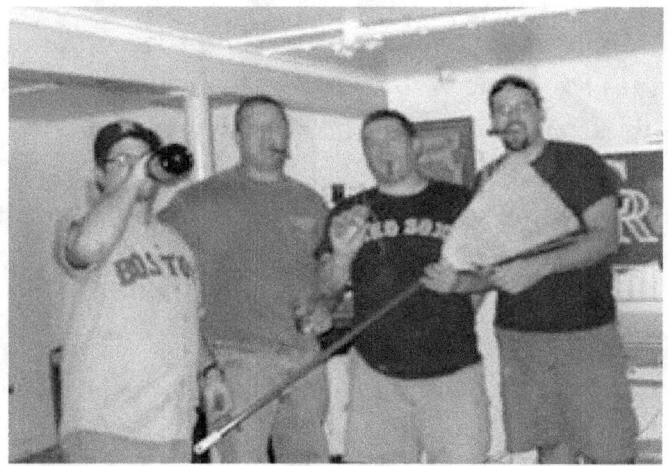

f'ing dave

Early on, my friend Fred visited and had a message from another friend of ours in Texas who we don't see as often as we like. Because we all share the dark humor that comes from this crazy thing called life, my friend Dave stated to Fred, "put a pillow over his face." These are the friends I treasure – those friends, I guess, who will say the most ridiculous thing just to get a rise out of you. These are the guys that beat the shit out of you at your bachelor party. The ones you get in trouble with are the ones you treasure for the rest of your life.

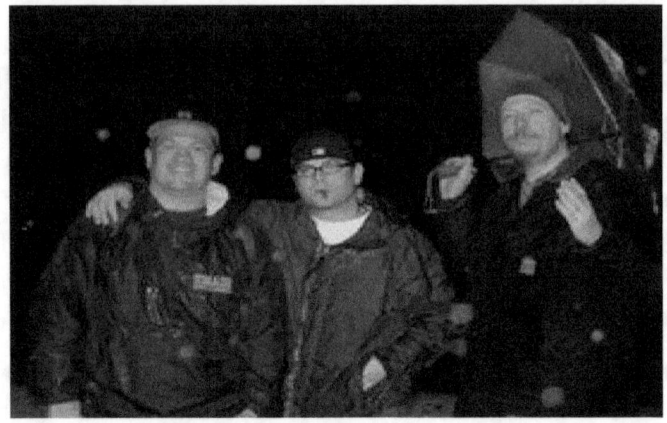
shea Astaire

People kept coming and coming -- close friends, family, colleagues Everyone would come. I had so many guests, one of the front desk people at Spaulding stated "this guy gets more visitors than the Pope." Everyone went out of their way to come see me. Everyone brought a little bit of the quilt that I call my crazy life.

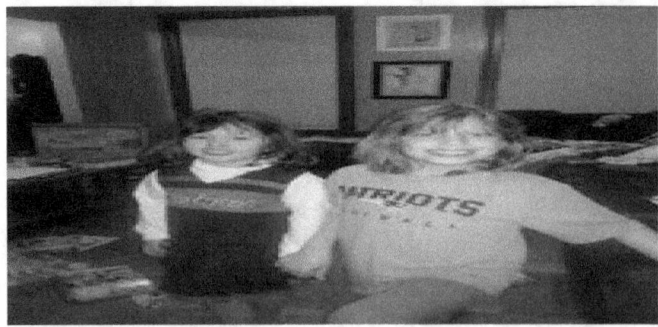

Your kids are essential visitors. If my wife was visitor number one – the straw that stirs the drink, the Reggie Jackson of my team – my kids were 1.5 and 1.75, maybe like Mickey Rivers and Thurman Munson. (These Yankee references are killing me but there was only one man who truly stirred the drink and that was Reggie, and the fact that I can compare him to Becky again just makes me laugh inside which amuses me)

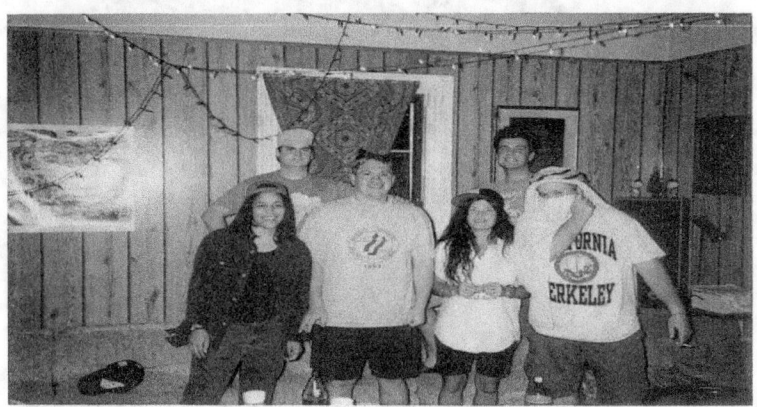

Many years ago when attending Framingham State and beyond that living in Somerville, I met a great number of people who would become near family to me. My Cameron crew was essential in this recovery. We've shared our ups and downs, our weddings, the births of our children and sadly the occasional funeral. Included in this group were a bunch of my boys. My boys would do anything for me and I for them. However, my girls are essential to me as well. In fact, other than my call to the paramedics to pick me up for the hospital, the only other person I called was Kathleen, knowing that she would be the only one who would be wicked pissed off if I did not call her, stroke be damned.

I'm going to make the mistake of calling out a couple other individuals because they really hit me at the right time. If there were some ultimate plan for me, you couldn't have had the timing any better than these visits.

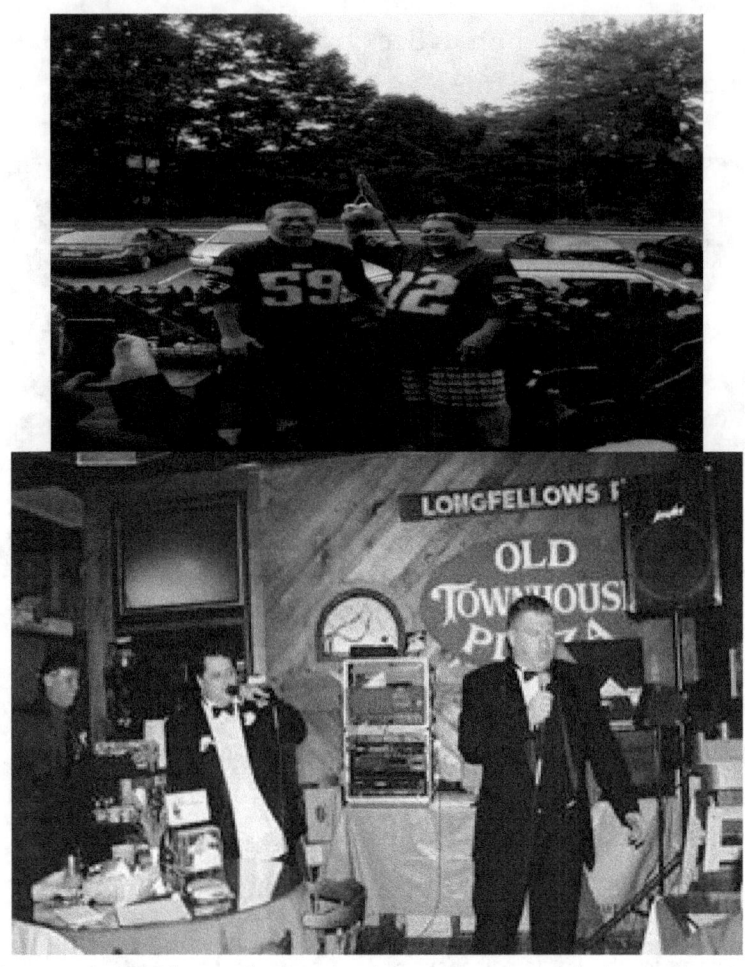

We are probably at the age where we shouldn't rank our friends. I mean it could just be a really big tie for first or second, but I can't say enough about my bestie, my ace boon, my brother Tim Taylor. Whenever something goes wrong, Clubba is there. And sometimes it's not even his fault.

Clubba has an eye for saying the right thing at the right time. Some people would argue he never stops talking so it's just dumb luck. I've known Tim since I was in intermediate school, but we became very close friends soon after high school. It was a case where my sister's best friend married my best friend, so we spend all our holidays together and shared pretty much every significant event in our lives. I treat his kids as my niece and nephew just as I treat my blood nieces and nephews and his wife. Well to be honest, if you asked my sisters they would say better than I even treat them. So that's the background.

Two Sundays in a row, Tim made the trip from the Cape to come and watch football with me. Both Tim and I can pretty much be found in the same place on Sundays, nursing a couple drinks on the couch watching football on television. Tim brought up stuffed quahogs and chowder at a time when I felt worthless and exhibited the friendship, brotherhood, and love that we built over a lifetime. Brother, I can never thank you enough. You seem to think that it was no big deal but it kept pushing my ass forward towards this point in my recovery. The same can be said for my sisters and mother but to be honest that's shit they're supposed to do. Not that I didn't appreciate it.

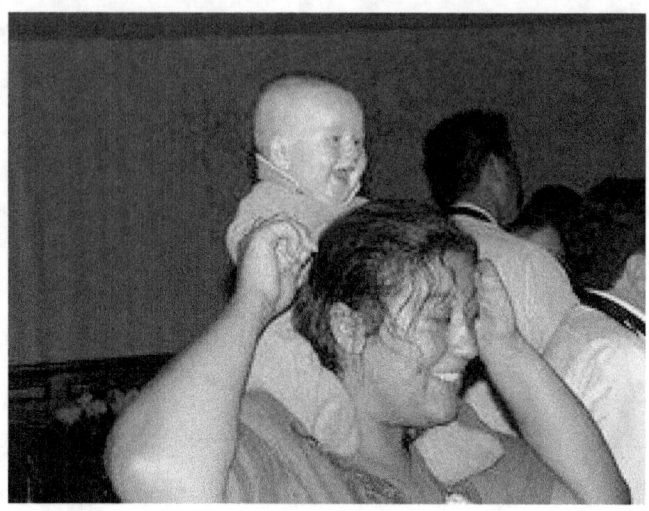

Julie, there's too much of Emma and Eneida in you and it's not like you had a choice.

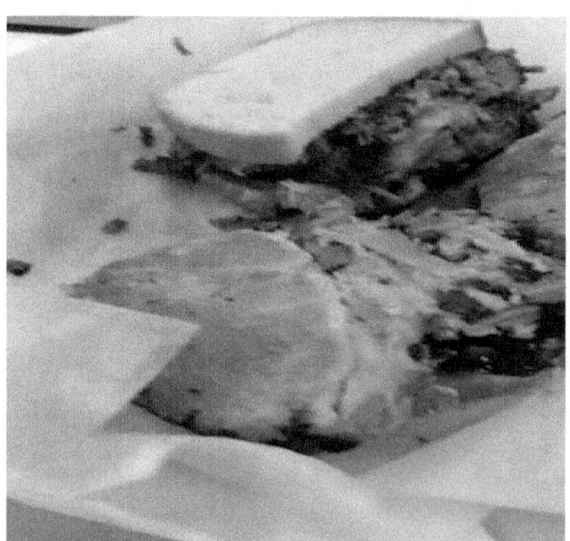

pastrami and corned beef on rye hell yeah

Although the sandwich my mother brought from Katz Deli was one of the best I ever had.

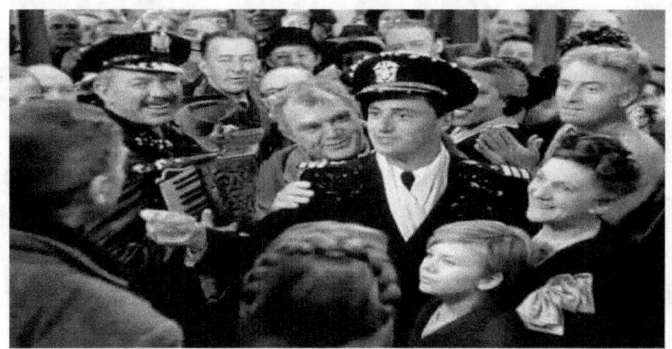

I also want to thank my friend Chez. The fool flew up in a blizzard ehrr drove from Virginia overnight. Fancy hotels aside, let's face it. The back of your car was probably great accommodations, but the thought and the visit meant the world to me. I've always admired your sense of loyalty, class and, of course, ridiculous skyhook in the paint. Again, I do not want to dismiss the efforts of my local friends who constantly made the trip over but y'all can face it, you are not Chez and you know this, man.

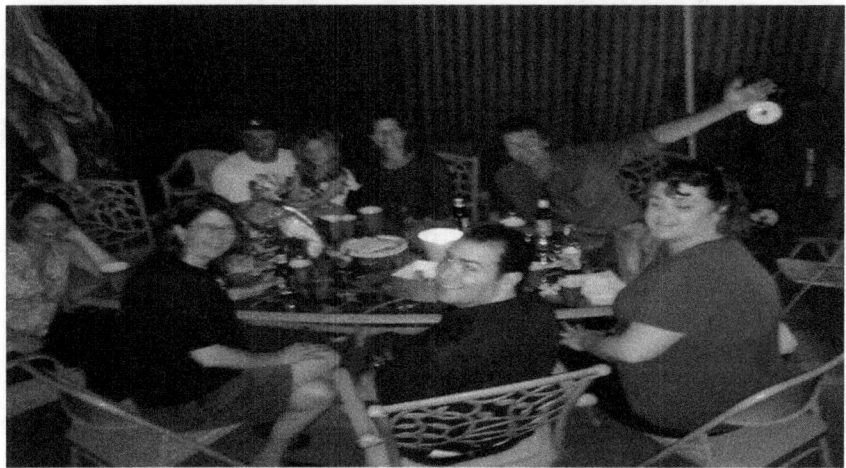

My coworkers, colleagues and friends made multiple visits to ensure me that the work I found so important was being completed and that the work of the team was moving without a hitch. To Bob, who came in and talked at length about the complexities of measurement for low-skilled students on the 10th grade MCAS, it was invigorating while at the same time helping me sleep thinking about it. To all my ESE friends, you are true public servants, doing the most you can do to support student learning and success. All bureaucratic jokes aside, you are pillars of our Republic.

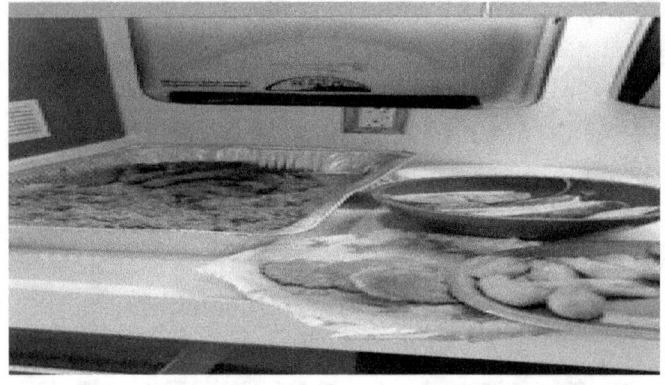

I can't say enough about my tio Miguel and my cousin Frances. Many of you don't know, but I took a lot of my parenting style from Miguel. He was always tough on his kids but was always present and always showed them love. I'll always remember that. Recently though they also came up from Virginia with restorative comidas via Holyoke. Those chuletas, arroz con gandules and tostones were magical. After eating plain hospital food as the majority of my diet, this Puerto Rican food brought me back home, or at least home in my heart. Certainly my doctors probably wouldn't have been too excited if I ate like this every day, but as far as spirits go it helped move me on my way to being regular Nyal.

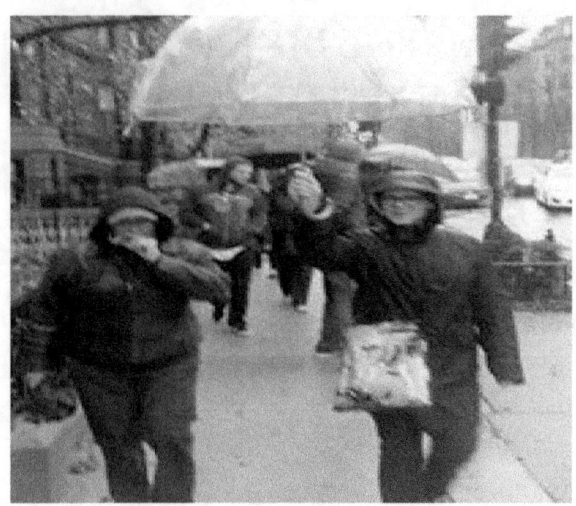
flask alley

So this is my quick and dangerous foray into gratitude for my support system. I tried to capture the spirit of a positive attitude in an earlier entry. The foundation of this positive attitude would have been crushed if I did not have the love, prayers, hope, laughs and attitudes of everyone who supported me both in person and in the rest of the world.

Enough cannot be said about those who watched my children, helped them have some joy and fun in what must've been a terrible situation for them, coworkers of my wife who supported all her efforts, those that completed a lot of chores around my house, whatever ridiculous project that I had going on and helped prepare my home for my eventual return. I did not hit on every highlight and at times was not the best host but I assure you that future visits to my home will be more complete with food, drink and joy.

BABY STEPS: THE BIKE RIDE AND RECREATIONAL THERAPY

Now get this
Oh (I know) you gonna take me home tonight (Please)
Oh down beside that red firelight
Are you gonna let it all hang out?
Fat bottomed girls you make the rockin' world go round yeah
Fat bottomed girls you make the rockin' world go round

Get on your bikes and ride
Ooh yeah oh yeah them fat bottomed girls
Fat bottomed girls
Yeah yeah yeah
Alright, ride 'em, c'mon
Fat bottomed girls, yes yes
Queen

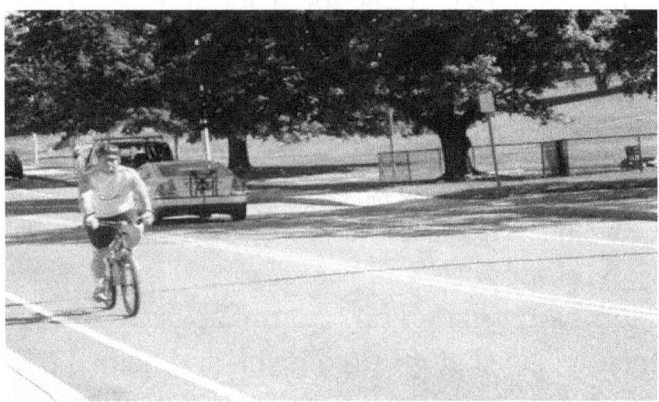

in more mobile days

One of my favorite events of the year is the Tufts floating hospital Cycle for Life. As many of you know, every year for the past eight years we've put together a team to ride for Tufts floating. I would never consider myself a cyclist, too chubby to wear spandex and terrified of skinny wheeled bikes and the inherent flats that come with them. Our team, *the Worst Peloton Ever,* rides a 25-mile ride and has raised about $42,000 over the last eight years to support kids with cancer. None of us really trains for this event, but it's a lot of fun.

Initially, it really came out of my love of urban biking. Years ago I lived in Somerville, commuting by bicycle was not what it is now. It was something the kids did to get to school or perhaps new immigrants to work. I soon found it was the fastest way to get anywhere around town, and when I was a youth worker in Cambridge and later director of a program, I could get from site to site much quicker than walking or even taking the T. As the years went on it became my favorite recreational activity.

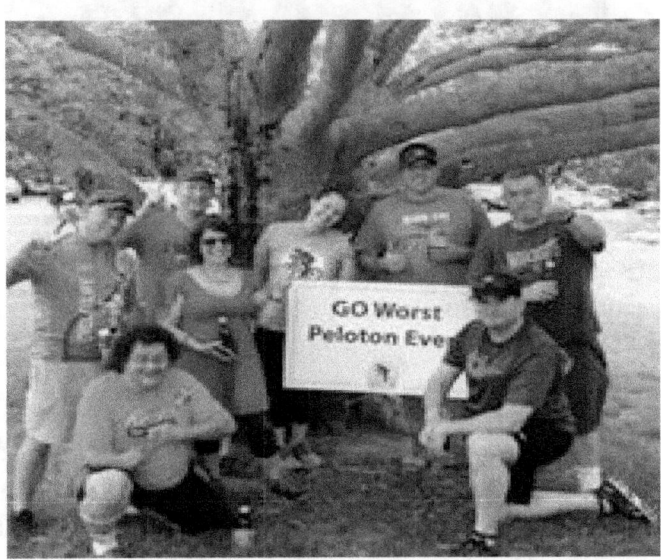

team 2016

When I was in rehab, as I have said there was a lot of focus on various forms of rehabilitation, most of which focused on specific weaknesses. In addition, Spaulding has something called recreational therapy. It seems that the theory behind recreational therapy was to use a host of these skills that you are trying to hone in on in a more recreational(duh), engaging and holistic environment. Recreational therapy hosted many different individual and group events.

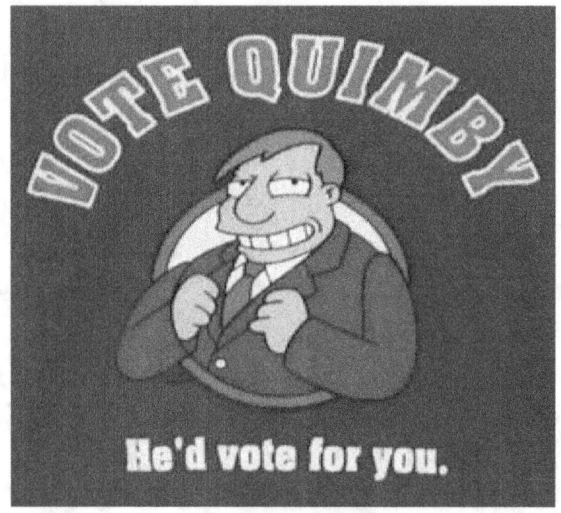

current events

One thing they also did was coordinate with the occupational therapists for our OT groups. When I was inside, I wanted to take advantage of every possible activity. Well, not every activity. I wasn't big on the therapy dogs, the beading classes, movies (the first movie they showed was *Concussion* for some godforsaken reason) or manicures. However, I was on board for most of the groups, classes, and any other opportunities that would assist my recovery.

Part of this was just for any interaction with anyone, particularly other people who were stroke survivors. Parts of the OT group activities seemed very silly. We would play name games. Discussing current events was valuable, since for many of us each day just ran into the next one. Thankfully there was not so much conversation about current politics (for those who are reading this afterwards this was during the presidential campaign) but we talk about ourselves and our situations. Some of these were heartbreaking like the aforementioned woman who had a stroke, laid on the ground for two days before anyone noticed she was missing, and also had a cat dying of cancer. Some of this really works with your empathy skills and, as a younger person who frankly did not have the other health issues that many of these older folks had, I felt blessed.

The part of these sessions that related to recreational therapy were the things that were silly but actually kind of fun. We played corn hole, a modified form of table hockey and even something I thought I would hate – music therapy – which is not as annoying as I expected. I made a couple buddies in the sessions but it is not like we would hang out in each other's rooms.

Most of the stay in a hospital is fairly solitary. I had tons of visitors and therapists and nurses and doctors, but for the most part as a "crip" 90% of my time spent with norms. I so wish this were different. I met a couple cool cats in these sessions, particularly some younger folks I would've liked to spend more time with. The other day, in fact, I was lucky enough to run into a stroke survivor at MGH at my neurologist appointment. His name was O'Neil and he had a young son. I think even our limited time talking we bonded us as dads. I wish I had been able to talk a little more with him during this day. The real beauty though was when I saw him last week he was walking without a cane and you would never know he was a stroke survivor. In fact, it looked like he had transferred back into a norm. I also met a couple other folks, older folks, and I would say hi and give them a smile in the gym, I felt it was part of my function at rehab to be the upbeat guy.

Outside of the group, recreational therapy provides other services. I had never even heard of such a thing. Leah was the director of the program and she had an intern from UNH named Jamie. They went over a host of opportunities for recreational therapy; some of them were less complex, play the Wii or other activities that involved hand eye coordination. One afternoon they invited me downstairs and asked me what type of activity I wanted to do. Among the choices were corn hole outside right along the mystic and catch with a Velcro ball and glove. I chose this for the opportunity to be was outside and feel a bit human. These silly sounding games actually helped with balance and strength and control, but mostly just for a few minutes you didn't feel like you are in the hospital. A burger and a beer could almost make you feel like you are outside at a barbecue enjoying a Saturday.

Recreational therapy also offers programming to what is called the adaptive sports program. Leah went over a series of options. She is trying to do the hard sell, so to speak, on sailing and kayaking on the mystic. I thought she was freaking crazy; there is no damn way life preservers be damned that I was going to go in the water with the bad arm and leg and unable to swim. She then told me a bit about the cycling program. I was very excited to do this as I had seen the recumbent bikes downstairs. Molly, my PT goddess, had said they can set up those bikes for people of all abilities. The first ride I got to participate in was a group ride. It seemed like most of the people had more ability than I did at this point, although I would learn shortly that some of them didn't quite have it all together cognitively and we would leave them behind a bit.

Spaulding has an entire adaptive sports group and staff. Their focus extends past cycling and the boating aspect to more complex activities for outpatient therapy. In addition, they work with schools that have students with disabilities to expand their opportunities to access sports. Gingerly, I was transferred from my wheelchair to the seat of the recumbent bike. I spoke to the leader of the group about how excited I was to eventually get back on a real bike.

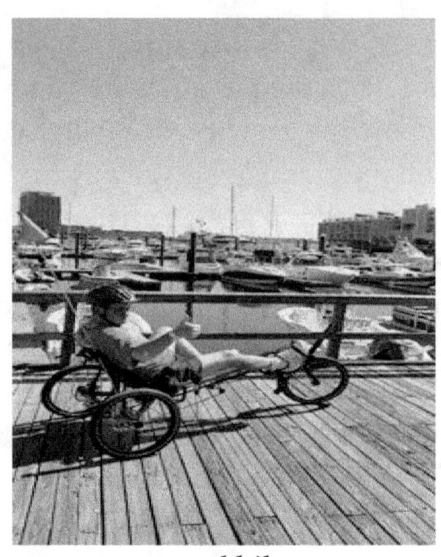

a real bike

She retorted with sort of a sneer "this is a real bike." At this point my right leg and arm were fine, they were as good as normal, but my left arm had virtually no strength or grip. My left leg was regaining strength but had a tendency to just flop around. They deftly Ace bandaged my hand into one grip and my left foot to the pedal. Essentially the bike could be controlled with just a right hand, both steering and brake.

I quickly got the hang of it and started moving forward. I wasn't going that fast and going up even the slightest incline took a great deal of effort but was exhilarating. We rode along the water over a series of boardwalks and paths. It was all so very exciting. My OT, who was a pretty skinny but fit woman, managed to do the whole ride on arm bike, making sure that I did not misbehave by going too fast or basically making a run for community college station and home. That being said I actually never had my wallet during the whole stay so my T pass was nowhere to be found. I think that was intentional.

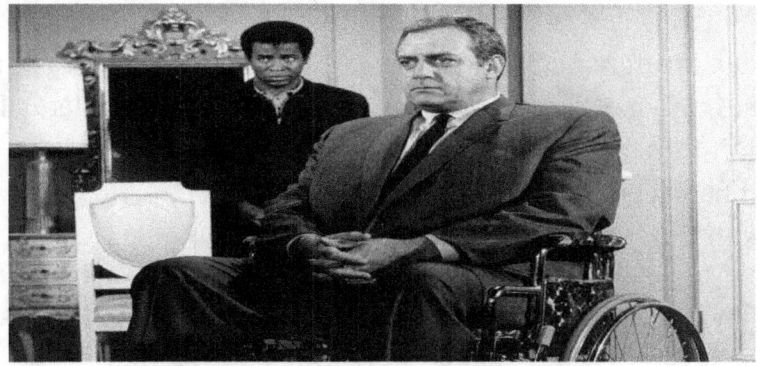
waiting for my next ride

Early the next week, I would get another opportunity to ride – this time with just staff. We went on a longer ride. I mean nothing crazy but up to the Charlestown Bridge and the locks. In this ride we went through the Navy yard and probably spent around 45 minutes cycling including a short time actually on the road. If given the opportunity to get outside and do something enjoyable, take it. If you want to feel like a regular guy again, riding a bike, looking at boats, and people watching really lifts your heart. Along with some of my key visitors, and the fortuitously timed Puerto Rican food, these rides really helped me to keep on keeping on.

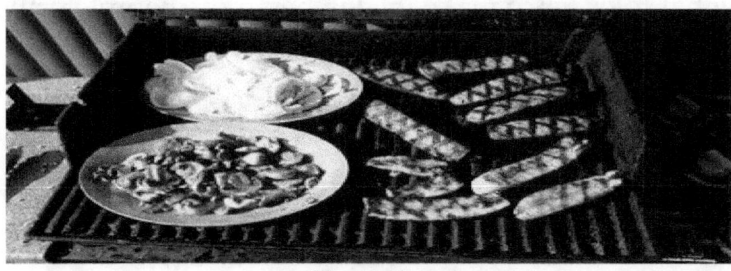
cooking at home

Another activity that was cosponsored between OT and recreational therapy was cooking. Erika and Leah said there may be a cooking group available. For those that know me, I can get kind of cranky in the kitchen. I have high expectations for cleaning as you go and being able to mise en place. Although I was with other stroke patients I didn't think it was best for me to be in a group. Most you that have cooked with me will realize I can be kind of a jerk in the kitchen, particularly when the potatoes are not peeled in time on Thanksgiving and I'm waiting on fucking Clubba to get his shit together. So they allowed me to cook alone. Well, that is, cook lunch for the therapists and my wife. I worked with the food they gave me and ended up making a sautéed chicken breast with peppers, onions and garlic. I was probably a couple items away from making a real nice Provençal chicken. The kitchen was in the model apartment on the stroke floor. The accommodations were kind of weak. It's all electric, of course, with probably the worst knives imaginable -- very dull and no good general chef's knife. For example, I was using a boning and paring knife to cut onions and peppers, cucumbers and make the salad. It wasn't about the meal itself, but the ability to do some of life's daily activities. I cooked a meal and served Becky and my therapists. All things considered it came out pretty well. (Leah later asked me what to order to make the kitchen more complete and I suggested a good chef's knife and tongs.)

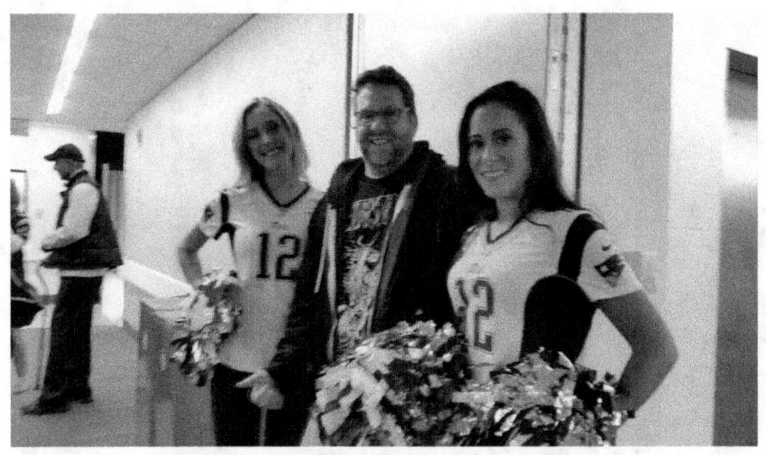
wow Davis what a surprise

Suddenly there was a knock on the door. It was my good friend Mike Davis who I had not seen since the stroke. This was his initial visit. Becky had worked to schedule visitors during the late afternoon time when I did not have any therapy. Mike was on his way to Maine and stopped by for the visit.

For those of you that know Davis he is often fortuitous in his timing. Just as I finished cooking the meal, we had a visit from some New England patriot cheerleaders and the Patriots mascot. It was just Davis' luck – there are women around and Mike shows up. Those of you who know Davis accept that things like this just happened. I fed Davis some chicken and then we went off to meet the Patriots cheerleaders that were visiting. It was sort of weird. These girls are super pretty but one of them was probably just a little taller than Elena and other than being curvier and athletic not that much bigger. It was especially creepier with some of the older gentleman. It was a nice break in the action and it just made for a good story.

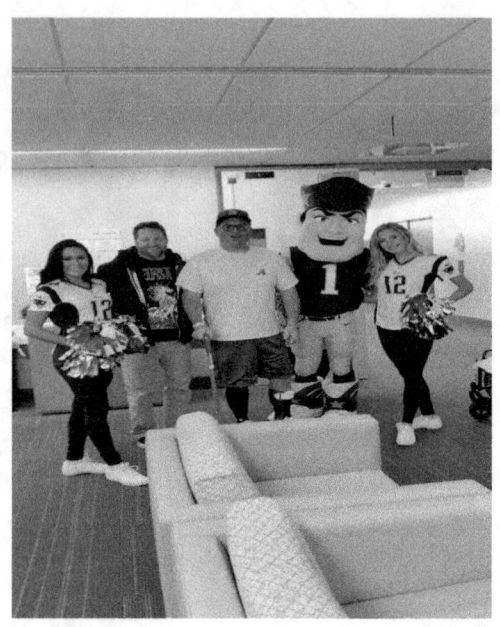

Another thing they really want you to do is go on what's called a community outing. Some of the community outings are somewhat mundane, like going grocery shopping or to Dunkin' Donuts. Others are more complex, such as apple picking or a visit to the zoo. My event, which felt like a final test, was to go out to lunch at Assembly. For those of you unfamiliar with Assembly, it is sort of a shopping district/almost planned community in Somerville. There are some outlets, a movie theater, a bunch of stores, housing, business properties and a ton of restaurants and bars. We were going out to lunch at a place called Wich. It should not surprise you that this was a sandwich joint. For this visit, I was going sans wheelchair for the first time over a long distance. With cane in tow and my wife and a few therapists, we went to the parking garage. I ambled over to the van and somehow climbed in the back. I'm not exceptionally tall but even at my height doing stuff like climbing and bending forward simultaneously were very difficult. It was the hardest part of the journey other than Molly making me carry my own drink at the restaurant and trying to sit on a high stool.

It was a fairly long walk. What I didn't realize was that the Spaulding vans, even though they were certain to have patients with disabilities, are not allowed to park in handicapped spaces. One thing about learning to walk again is that you understand why toddlers need naps. It is really exhausting. Apparently I did all right ambulating around Assembly but by the time I got back (as most of you who had a stroke or work with someone who had a stroke), even the most rudimentary basic activities are exhausting. I got back and slumped into my wheelchair.

For anyone in rehab, I recommend taking advantage of what's offered to you. No matter what your interest is, you are likely to find something to do and you may even want to stretch your interest somewhat. As I keep saying, you will not get better unless you get engaged in your own recovery. No one is going to recover you for you. It is based on effort and attitude to even get out of the hospital and on your way home. I don't know if I can keep up this attitude effort for the foreseeable future, but lying in bed or even a chair feeling sorry for yourself is going to get you nowhere. It may even frustrate the most patient and loving of families. Now, pray that I can keep it up.

PREPARE TO UNLOAD

Now that I escape, sleepwalker awake
 Those who could relate know the world ain't cake
Jail bars ain't golden gates
 Those who fake, they break,
 When they meet their 400 pound mate
 If I could rule the world
 Everyone would have a gun in the ghetto of course
 When giddyupin' on their horse
 I Kick a rhyme drinkin' moonshine
 I pour a sip on the concrete, for the deceased
 But no don't weep, Wyclef's in a state of sleep
 Thinkin' 'bout the robbery that I did last week.
 Money in the bag, banker looked like a drag
 I want to play with pelicans from here to Baghdad
 Gun blast, think fast, I think I'm hit
 My girl pinched my hips to see if I still exist.
 I think not, I'll send a letter to my friends,
 A born again hooligan only to be king again.
The Fugees

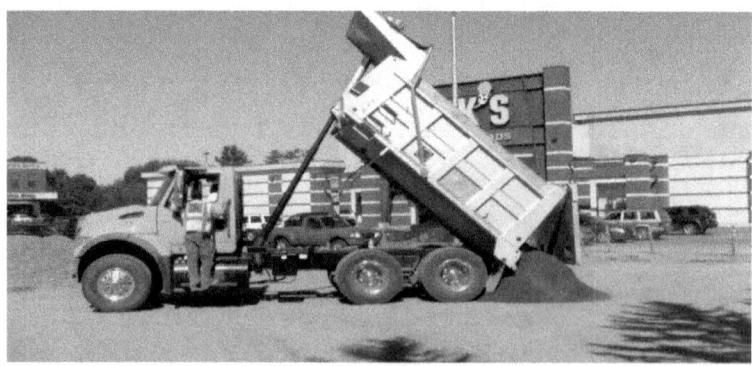

Many chapters start out with some song lyrics that may or
may not reflect what is in the actual posting. Most of my

life, I walk around with a soundtrack in my head. I found it to be mentally balancing to get me through the day. Sometimes the songs are just jingles, sometimes a little more complex.

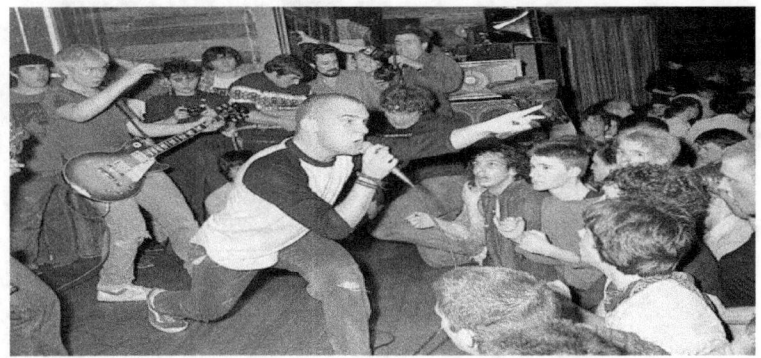

These songs get me through good days and bad days. Sometimes it is as simple as "here comes Nyal, he's one tough customer" which I stole from Randall in Clerks. Other times it will be the entire discography of Minor Threat or the entire album of the Clash, Sandinista. It assists me when I write at work and helps to increase my vocabulary beyond acronyms, jargon and hackneyed business conversation. I wonder if other people do this. I am often tempted to go up to them and say "what's the last song you were thinking of."

[This will be one of the last two or three blogs that is written in the past tense, after this very therapeutic blast in the first week of posting, I will likely slow down to maybe once a week. The change in my physical abilities has become somewhat incremental, I mean it's getting better, but I'm not sure enough to write about. But we'll see because I don't return to work part time until November 14 so this is a good cognitive exercise as well as being inspirational to me to tell a story that hopefully others will be able to use as a foundation for recovery or to help others recover.]

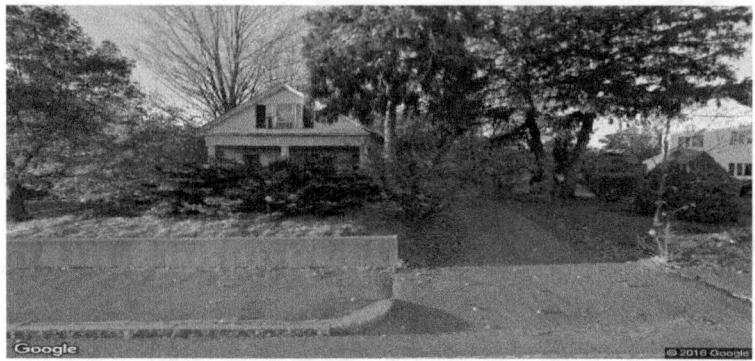

108 in Framingham

When we lived in Framingham for a time in an awesome but somewhat messy and crazy house we had a street sign that Tim or someone had acquired that said "prepare to unload" in our downstairs bathroom. For some reason as I was getting ready to leave, perhaps because of my continuing difficulty using the restroom without assistance, I kept thinking about the sign and just how ridiculous it was, as I see much of my life in general. Along with music, flashbacks of funny things in the past constantly flow through my head. I have to also say I tend to also relive all the fuck ups that I've had in my life as well and unfortunately regret them and wish I could've done better. Getting to Spaulding was a huge victory. The prospect of leaving Spaulding was even better.

There's no place like home, particularly for me. I don't really enjoy vacations that I have to travel to. We've designed our home to fit pretty much all of our daily needs, so why the hell would I want to go anywhere else?

So I was anxious to get home despite my continuing lack of mobility and physically how much easier it was to be in Spaulding. People bring you food, whisk you off to appointments; in general, your life is managed either by your family or the staff there.

In preparation for leaving, there were many things that had to be done. I never was officially told what my release day was. The general aspect of rehab is that your insurance really controls the length of your stay. I was pretty happy to have really good insurance, so that didn't seem to be an issue. My speech pathologist leaked to me one day that my release date was October 4. I don't remember officially hearing that from anyone in any specific declaration but it became known to myself, my family and all the staff.

As I got to my last week, I actually started to get a little nervous – how would I be climbing the stairs, getting around the kids' toys, getting around the kids, using the two bathrooms and avoiding my cats below on the floor. This anxiety was, of course, tempered with the excitement of going home.

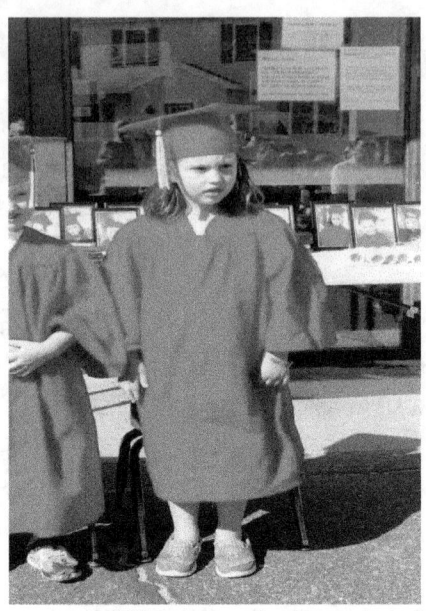
a different graduation

To get ready, they essentially would "graduate" me from physical and occupational therapy. Along with the previously mentioned exercises of the community outing and cooking in the kitchen, they also started to make sure I could transfer from toilet up and down and get into the shower safely with a shower chair using grab bars. My wife dutifully bought all the necessary home equipment.

This is an important part of your recovery. A week or so before you return home, have a detailed conversation with your therapist (they probably will initiate it anyway) about how your house is set up. If necessary, have someone take pictures of everywhere there is a possible physical transition such as stairs and other potential obstacles. You may need to have a friend or contractor help with grab bars in the shower and a railing like we did. We were lucky to have our friend Nick take care of all these issues. You will most likely want to have someone help clean the house. Many of my chores at home included cleaning and organizing, but unfortunately those that love you will have to step up for a while. At this point I was fairly strong. Other people will advance at a different pace and some will move on to skilled nursing before heading home.

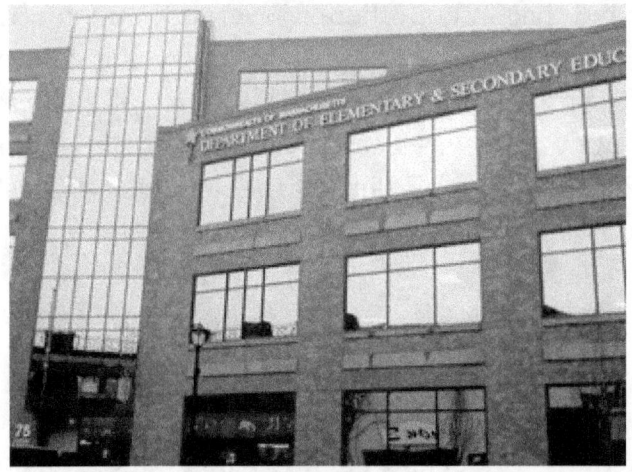
work

At this point I'm pretty anxious to get back to work, but not before filling out a "fitness to work" form along with your FMLA forms. Most of my work is knowledge work, involving intellectual stamina, communication, data analysis and sometimes dealing with difficult people. As part of my exit I had a neuropsych exam. This exam helps to quantify your cognitive readiness to return to life and work. There are no Rorschach tests or laying on a couch talking about your mother. It's more about how your brain is working around memory and other cognition. It's very similar to what you are working on in speech pathology. In fact, some of the exercises are identical and some you may have memorized.

It's a long exam. It can take up to three hours or more with a psychologist asking you a series of questions. Initially there are some questions about your attitude and general psychological well-being. They'll ask you questions about yourself that are quite personal, around drug use, family life and things of that nature but at this point you're likely to have put that shit out there to everyone and you're somewhat comfortable talking about it even if you're somewhat private person. I don't want to call the test grueling but there was a certain amount of stamina needed to complete the tests and in fact that is part of the test; can you keep thinking, remembering and completing all the exercises.

Some are very difficult and, in my case and probably many of yours, they see what level you're on. If you dropped out of elementary school and got no further education the test will be structured somewhat differently than those with advanced degrees. I did pretty well on these tests and got to the point that I was joking around with the psychologist. One of the stories identified State Street as being in South Boston, which I pointed out was incorrect. He laughed and indicated just go with the story and memorizing it. I told him, well it goes beyond my best instincts but I'll do it just so I can pass this test. After the test was over he indicated to me that I did well but that a much longer report would be developed. He later came back and went over the results. This part is important if you plan to return to work in a fairly rapid manner. You don't have to release all the results. For example, there is no reason for HR to know how much I smoked pot as a teenager and young man, but there is an executive summary that is very helpful.

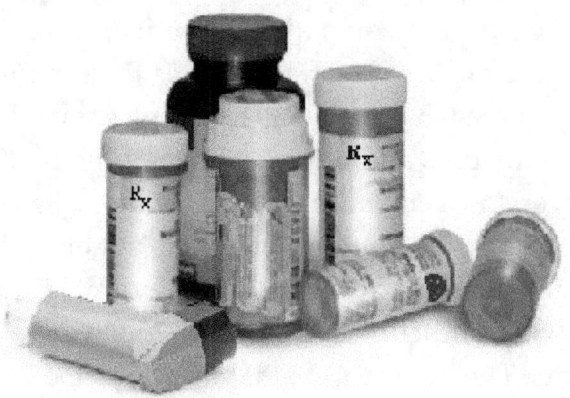

I was very excited to leave despite my anxiety about being safe when I returned home. They also take time to review your meds. I was taking no medication at all before my stroke although I probably should have but that's another story. Getting used to taking these medications and my old own blood pressure twice a day would take some effort. During your entire stay, the nurses drill you on your medications, some of them are very difficult to pronounce but you get to the point that you got them down, those in the morning and those at night. For the rest of my life I will probably take high blood pressure medication and anti-cholesterol medication even though my cholesterol was not even that high.

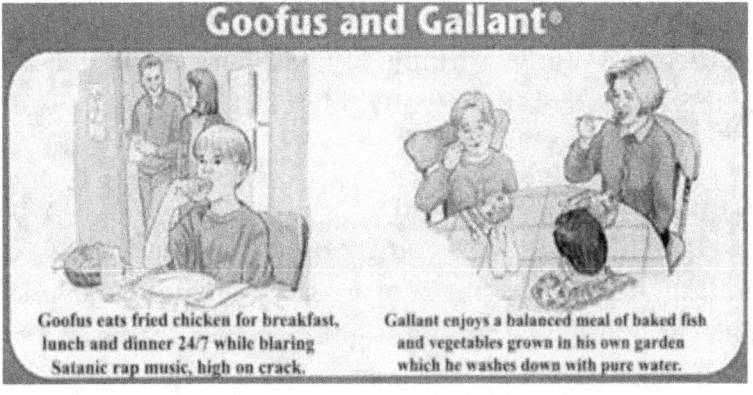

Goofus and Gallant®

Goofus eats fried chicken for breakfast, lunch and dinner 24/7 while blaring Satanic rap music, high on crack.

Gallant enjoys a balanced meal of baked fish and vegetables grown in his own garden which he washes down with pure water.

Some of the stuff they do may seem ludicrous and very obvious but there are specific protocols to prepare you whether you are Goofus or Gallant. They showed me how to separate my pills and put them in the pillbox. They will go over every movement that you do in your daily activities, ask if you feel physically safe at home, i.e. will Becky beat me and remind me to stay hydrated, then back to their favorite functions, urinating and bowel movements. They tell you that if you pee blood or fall down the stairs, it is a good idea to call your primary care physician. Most importantly, they will help you schedule all your next appointments for the next few weeks or even months. As much as I joke around about some of the child-like treatment, I did understand and appreciate the help.

At Spaulding on Monday afternoons all the therapists meet with the doctor who is treating you. They discuss your progress or lack thereof and determine when you are leaving. Once again I wasn't privy to those meetings and my case manager didn't communicate the results very well (albeit she was a very nice lady). It is important for you and whoever is managing your care for your family to always show the initiative of asking lots of questions. I'm a strong believer in the fact that there are stupid questions, I hear the most of my working day. But here, it's better to be safe than sorry and they really don't mind.

Getting ready to leave felt like the same anxiety I felt when I was laying on Clubba's couch on the morning of my wedding. It was the irrational anxiety that you get even when you know everything is going to be just fine and it will be. This preparation to go home is as essential as going home itself.

HOME

This place always gets to me like an old familiar song,
 Stirring up old feelings that I thought were long gone.
 I guess that you can move away but you cannot escape where
you're from.

 Home, nothing ever changes.
 Home, and I wouldn't want it to.
 Home, everything's the same as I left it when I went away to
make myself anew.

 The old familiar wallpaper and a battered old settee,
 The china doll that dad brought back from the war in Germany,
 The faintest smell of creosote and a cup of milky tea,
 This is home
Billy Bragg

Take me down
 To the paradise city
 Where the grass is green
 And the girls are pretty
 Oh, won't you please take me home
Guns 'n' Roses

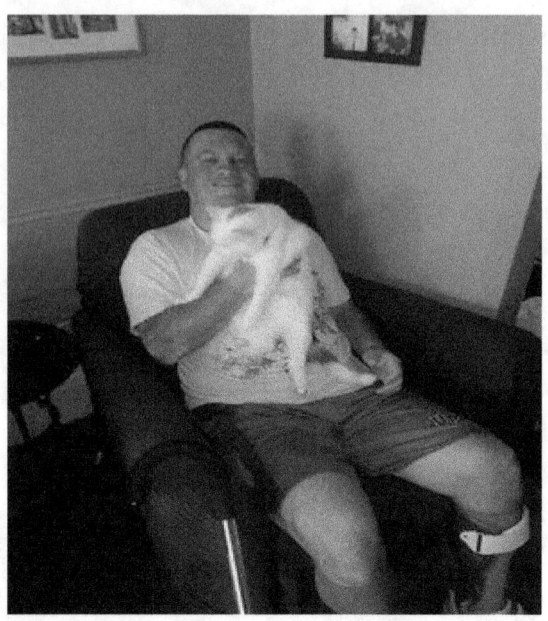

This entry really needed two sets of lyrics. The first song is off Billy Bragg's last album *Tooth and Nail*. This album was one of those cases where I really felt the artist grew up alongside of me, with the more revolutionary lyrics of youth and the more grown-up/dad lyrics of middle-age and being a productive family member. The second song which is as most you know Guns and Roses really just makes you want to drink beers and be in a mosh pit with friends. In the soundtrack of my life all these artists and bands are important.

In my previous entry I talked a bunch about getting ready to go home – about how much I love being home, how much I love to have my family fill its halls and my friends fill these rooms with fun, love, and joy. But there was anxiety at the prospect of going home. As I said, I guess Spaulding was easy. I had my last breakfast in bed the morning of Tuesday, October 4. I really didn't want another breakfast in bed until Father's Day, if then. My anxiety of not being in Spaulding was the fear that I wouldn't keep up the real physical progress I had made under the direction of my nurses and therapists. That I would step on the cat and fall down the stairs or trip over a shopkin or just have Mimi walk in front of me and have us both collapse on the floor -- which you know if you have kids would be entirely my fault.

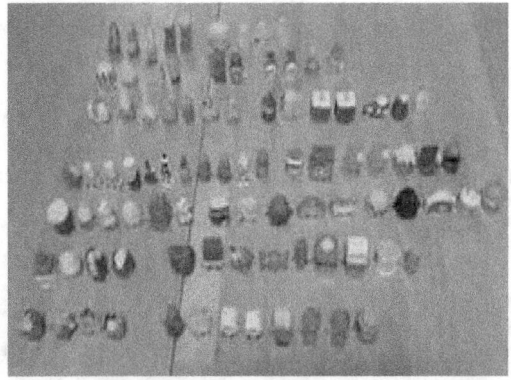

these are shopkins for the unaware

A quick play-by-play. The day before I was to leave they began to give me information about discharge, but not that much about discharge. I was still sort of confused. On top of that, I was called about participating in a research project around arm recovery after stroke, where the assessment would take three hours on the day I was supposed to leave. My motivation was that my occupational therapist, Erika, who was so helpful to me during my stay, was involved in the study. I am anything if ungrateful for her help and support.

The day before I had told Christina, my nurse, about this plan. To quote her "that's bullshit. They've had three weeks to assess you. Don't let them delay you from being discharged." (Don't say these ladies weren't in my corner)

On Tuesday morning, the project people came early to get my assessment done before my release. It was sort of the standard stroke assessment that I had already done about three dozen times, again to the point that I think I could give the assessment. These were different people than Erika, but we managed to get it done fairly quickly and I was prepared for release by 10 a.m. which was my scheduled discharge time.

The whole release was sort of anticlimactic. After being cared for, shepherded around, and scheduled, basically I was cut off the hook, ready to swim on my own. One of the aides I became friendly with offered to wheel me down to the lobby, mostly because she wanted to get off the floor. I did have a chance to give hugs to my nurse that was there, Christina, and all three of my therapists in appreciation for all they had done. I'm not sure if they understood the depths of my compliments and respect about how much they had done for me during my stay. If they are reading this or if you are a physical, occupational, or speech therapist, I'm not sure you realize how much impact you have on the beginning of the recovery for your patients.

After being dropped off in the lobby, Rebecca and I ambulated to her car. I still couldn't walk very well even with a cane. I had not been in a regular car in a month. Nonetheless, we were free! I won't be able to drive for a while but being in an automobile was really cool. I saw the route that everyone had taken to visit me over the past three weeks, which made me really appreciate those visitors.

Our first stop when returning the Melrose was at my barbershop. I was feeling a little shaggy. The good part about going to a regular barber is you never have to really talk to him unless you want. He never asked questions about how I want my haircut, he just shaves it down. Dave the barber is old school. The newspaper at the shop is the Herald and if Law and Order is not on the television, it's strange. Today, for some reason Match Game 78 was on the television very loud. I asked use the restroom, and the toilet was full of cigarettes and the room just plain nasty. Thus, my introduction into a non-sterile, non-hospital environment was pretty stark.

My first day home was a little shaky as everything is not hospital safe. Getting up the stairs was fairly easy having the railing to balance me, but that last step in the house was kinda hinky. There was nothing to grab onto and I had to work on faith. Even with some poor cane placement and a left leg that might not want to cooperate, we got in the house where I saw my friends' handiwork and help to get the house together. Again, counting my blessings.

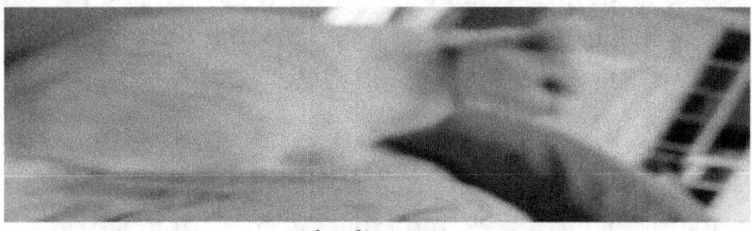

healing cat

The first day home was awesome but challenging, however my able wife and angelic brats guided me through. We ordered Thai food, got to watch random things on my big television, got to sit in my comfy chair and, with the assistance of my white cat purring, made it through the day. The First day on this journey I was running on smiles and hugs with hopes of being back to grumpy Nyal as soon as possible.

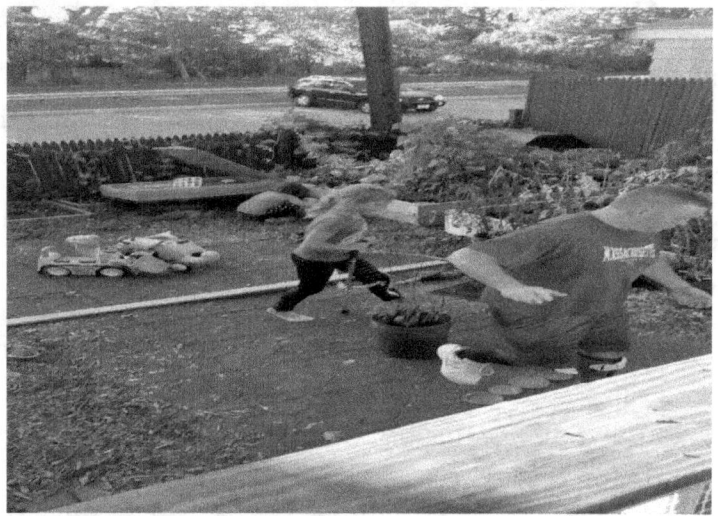

Finally, I got an opportunity to visit my backyard, to see my garden. Due to the weather it was in its last throes, but still contained a ton of green beans. Basically, the tomatoes were gone. Getting those last few tomatoes are always kind of depressing, realizing that for the next nine months you will be eating something that are called tomatoes but have no relation to what is picked fresh off the vine.

I also engaged with my PT assistant, Elena, to set up some simple obstacle courses in the backyard to practice on mobility. I even managed to have a little sword fight with

Marisol. These are some of the small things you miss. I always knew I was their dad and their father in the hospital. They were very frequent visitors and we could talk about our days and how well they were doing in school. However, it wasn't until this moment – the simple playing around – where I was Papa again. Although not as mobile, the fun-loving guy fussing around his babies, laughing together and just doing stupid shit just makes my heart warm. Now all the work around recovery was at this point just to get into this half-hour in my backyard. Let me say that I appreciate every blessing that has been given to me in my life, and as much as my kids are often ungrateful pains in the ass, I love them unconditionally with every depth of my heart.

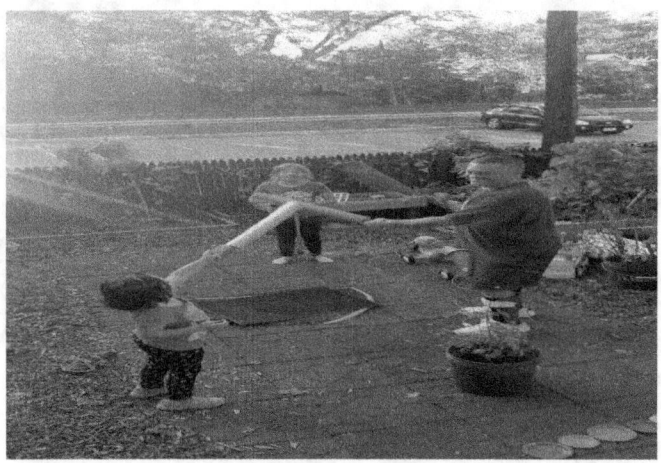

no holds barred

The first couple nights I slept better than in the hospital but still not very well. I still had to use the urinal bedside as in the middle of the night it was quite a process to get to the bathroom due to another weird step on top of our stairs and the restroom. Almost immediately I began to develop a little bit of independence. Nick had set the shower grab bars perfectly for use, so very quickly I became almost 100% independent in the bathroom. You don't know how good that feels. Yeah, the toothpaste could be a little challenge, but I was even putting in my own contact lenses which made me feel a lot better.

A day or two later we made a quick visit to the Stoneham zoo – only for about 45 minutes. Of course, Marisol was upset because we didn't have enough time to play in the playground. In her mind, everything should just be normal again. I did get a good chance to walk with my family, albeit slow and with a cane, the way a family should do things – enjoying their time together, despite your younger daughters whining.

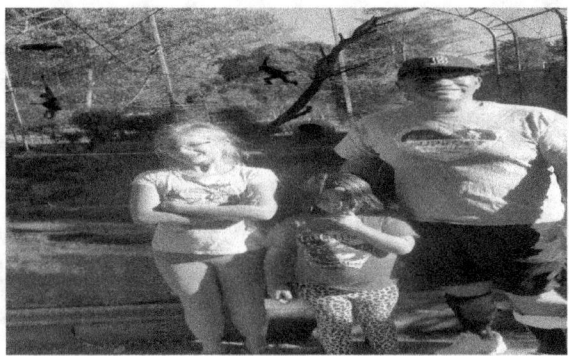
the gibbons

I'm not perfect yet, nor will I ever be perfect. I still haven't seen my beloved basement but the huge step of going over that doorstep is a victory over this stroke.

ADAPTATION

A smash of glass and the rumble of boots
An electric train and a ripped-up phone booth
Paint-splattered walls and the cry of a tomcat
Lights going out and a kick in the balls

I say that's entertainment
That's entertainment
La la la la la, ah
La la la la la, ah

Days of speed and slow-time Mondays
Pissing down with rain on a boring Wednesday
Watching the news and not eating your tea
A freezing cold flat with damp on the walls

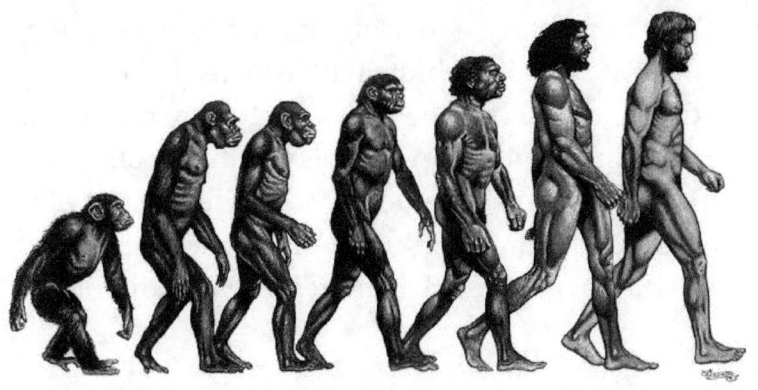

Going home is sort of like getting married – you have a great time, it's a great memory but then the actual marriage begins. Any type of relationship requires work, patience, occasional frustration and, of course, great fun and joy. I'm trying to personify what it is to adjust getting home after a stroke. The journey after crossing the threshold is twisty and curvy.

Everything is really different. Everything I saw -- my bicycle, my car, looking down the basement stairs, and visiting my yard really illustrated things I would not be able to do for a while. As much as my life was becoming more "normal" it was going to be a long time before I got anywhere close to 100%.

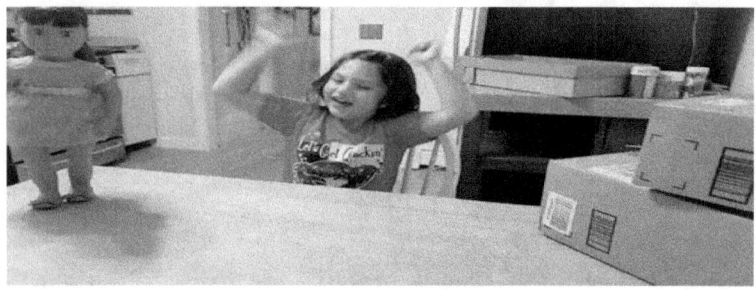

One of my goals when I was in rehab was to get to Marisol's birthday party -- to actually walk in as her Papa, eat cake and pizza and celebrate with friends and family like any decent dad should be able to. Saturday the eighth, just four days after my release, I achieved that goal. Fortunately, it was at the Malden YMCA which has pretty good access. Automatic doors and ramps make things much easier for even those that are temporarily disabled.

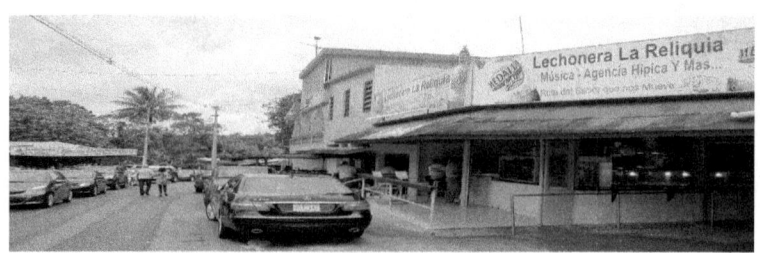

GUAVATE THE HAPPIEST PLACE ON EARTH

Years ago when I was in Puerto Rico with my grandfather sort of chauffeuring him around the island, I really got to know how important ADA was for America. Puerto Rico while an associated Commonwealth of the United States had not really caught up with ADA (at least at that point). With buildings that were over 500 years old, most did not have the access you would have for someone who is disabled. My grandfather suffered a stroke and could sorta move around but mostly was confined to this three-wheel electric lark type vehicle. I would race behind him on foot around the streets of San Juan, Cayey, Ponce and everywhere on the island you could possibly imagine. This is when I started to discover how much stairs and other obstacles could deny access to folks, mostly because I would hump that stupid machine over curbs into cars and everywhere else you could possibly imagine. You also really learn to appreciate ramps and such after you have kids and are pushing them in the stroller.

Mine appears to be somewhat of a temporary disability. I'm much more able than I was and if you saw me at a restaurant or even walking around the mall or the street you'd probably just imagine that I'd had a leg injury, knee replacement or something of that nature and not major brain trauma. Adjusting to the world is hard. I liked being active and I want to do stuff, which sometimes can be frustrating. It can take me close to 25 minutes to shower and get dressed for the day, even though it's just shorts, a T-shirt and shoes and socks. Ordinarily it would take 10 to 15. I can't do simple things like clean the cat box or fish tank. Doing dishes with the dishwasher, loading and unloading would be a real effort. I was used to doing a considerable amount of the housework, which now falls on my wife, along with everything else to bear the burden.

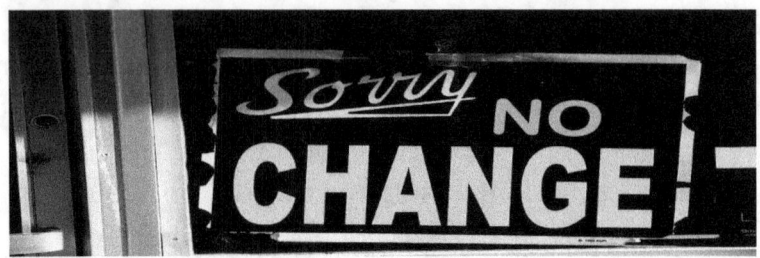

Although I'm progressive, ironically I don't like change very much. As my friend Chez would say "some call it a rut, I call it a groove." My days before the stroke were usually planned out -- get ready, get the kids to school, work, pick up kids, play or do work around the house, play on the Internet or watch TV or read and then go to sleep. Weekends would differ but would always require a lot of activity, particularly around my puttering around the house or working in the garden.

Not having a plan for the day is somewhat challenging. Checking blood pressure, taking meds, things that you were doing in the hospital but are now responsible for, become a big part of your job. When it comes down to it, I will have missed nearly 10 weeks of work (all of which are being paid for) and sorta be out of the loop with the real world. The idea of the real world is kind of funny. Nothing has been more real to me in my life other than the birth of my children than this stroke yet it is not really tied to the outside world. As much as been done for me and continues to be done, the responsibility of recovery is going to fall on me.

Initially upon release, I was assigned home care that consisted of visits from occupational therapy, physical therapy and, at one point, even a nurse because I was considered homebound. The occupational therapy and physical therapy at home is much different than that in the hospital or even the upcoming outpatient therapy. There is no opportunity to use machines or other devices and most of it is really making sure you're following through with your exercises. It is very easy to start skipping your exercises when no one is watching. By nature, and evolution most humans do the least they can to get by. Not everyone, but most of us normal folks are non-type A people. You gotta keep it up. You've got to do it on your own, but now, particularly with occupational therapy, I tend to cut corners. The therapists are very helpful in making sure you're keeping up with your schedule.

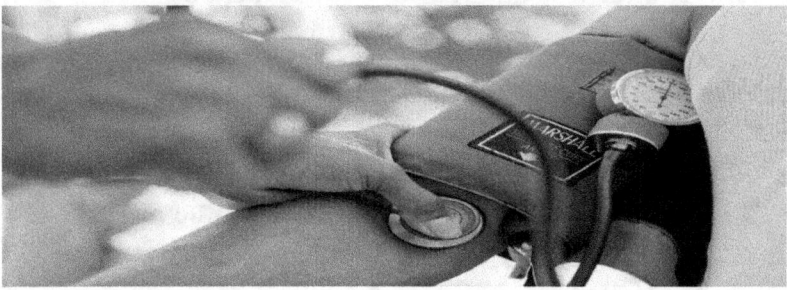

The Thursday after I was released, yes a mere 48 hours, my occupational therapist came in and took my blood pressure. She noted it was high and suggested I go to the emergency room. Becky wasn't here, it was just me and the therapist. Becky was at a PTO meeting at school and as soon as I texted her, she left the meeting. My occupational therapist had insisted that I go to the emergency room and, in fact, said if my wife did not arrive soon, she was going to call an ambulance. Obviously this probably made blood pressure go up even more. She also suggested that I not go to a local hospital but instead go to MGH directly.

Becky came home, our friend Andy diligently came over to watch the kids and we headed off. Again I'm going to escape any tough guy veneer that I have and tell you that I was sobbing. After two days at home the last thing I wanted was to be readmitted to the hospital. I had it so in my rearview even this quickly that I cannot imagine being incarcerated again. We showed up at MGH and were greeted by very friendly and helpful security guards who offered me a wheelchair. I sneered "no fucking way" but he insisted on walking by my side to the hospital. It made me think what it must be like to work in a hospital and be greeted by people who are sometimes at their worst even though they do really appreciate the help. In the hospital waiting room I was again asked about a chair. At this point I just told her I was fine. The wait wasn't that bad, but I did tell Becky that I need to get a sword cane so I could stab people that were completely irritating, such as one of the family members of someone who was waiting in the waiting room. Later in the week I wanted that sword cane to stab someone in the neck who was wearing a make America great hat at a diner. So another piece of advice: do not get a sword cane because you're easily irritable after a stroke.

Anyways, I was called by the nurse who took my blood pressure which was high 140/100 but not dangerously high. Sometimes you say just stupid things. I told one of the nurses, if I was admitted I was jumping out the window. Again don't say stuff like that -- it does no good.

But I was just being the way I am, you know, kind of a jackass. Soon the emergency physician saw us and we met for probably a total of 75 seconds. He told me unless I was peeing blood or having other stroke symptoms that I was fine. Unless my blood pressure went to 185/110 I should just stay home, relax and not get stressed out.

My blood pressure was stabilized but I still called my primary care physician, who assigned me another blood pressure pill. Since then I have the blood pressure of Uta Pippig. I'd never met my primary care physician. My old physician was changed, and while Dr. Taylor had bugged me to come in, I was waiting -- waiting to lose some weight and get healthier before I saw her so she would not hassle me. But here I am in stroke recovery coming in for my first visit. After so many visits, pokes, prodding, and piercing over the past five weeks, this visit was simple. She is very friendly, very pretty and did not yell at me or hassle me. We talked about meds, we talked about how my rehabilitation was going, and what my plan was for the near future.

Immediately I started talking about returning to work. I told her I was already working a little, nothing intense, just sharing ideas and giving advice to my coworkers. Because I passed all the cognitive tests, the main issues were that rehabilitation and my therapies had to come first. I had to make sure I was physically able to go back to work, to be able to safely move around the office and have the right accommodations for success.

Working for the state as I do is great as far as benefits and throughout the stroke HR has been super supportive. It doesn't hurt that one of the women in HR who is in charge of benefits is extremely helpful, kind, and competent. There is however, even for an experienced bureaucrat like me, an inordinate amount of paperwork to be completed which I still haven't finished. These are necessary to get the appropriate accommodations under ADA to do your job successfully. For me it is going to require an initial modification of my work schedule (being part-time and doing some work remotely) as well as speech-to-text software and likely limiting travel. This is an important part of your sanity as well. If you appreciate and value your work, you're gonna want to set a timeline for your return, so it doesn't feel like you're just floating around waiting for something magical to happen. Nothing is going to happen magically again. There is no reverse thunderbolt that can undo your stroke. It now becomes incremental, slow improvement. Other people, such as your therapist and friends, are going to notice these changes long before you do.

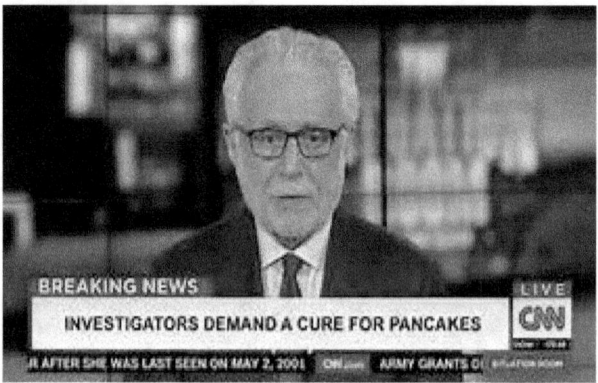

Another thing that I had to face was fatigue. Although I am starting to feel better, sleep better and even be a little more mobile, I continue to be exhausted even after a good night sleep. This seems strange due to my limited activity. I filled my time mostly with working on this chronicle, doing a little work and, for the first week and a half, re-watching The Wire. I wanted something that was stimulating and good that would not make me feel stupid.

I also made the mistake of watching CNN. It's incredible during this election campaign to realize how insipid much of the general public actually is and how much the media is willing to spoon-feed this population.

Fatigue is a hard battle and it's not depression, just true physical exhaustion. I've been told by others that much of this exhaustion is due to healing which is very tiring. It seems like every little thing just takes much more effort to be successful. I still get some visitors which is nice. I got to watch Tom Brady's comeback with friends and even enjoyed some nonalcoholic beer while watching the game. Well, I wouldn't say enjoyed since it kind of sucked -- the beer that is. I've taken another month off of any drinking because my balance is already screwed up. It's not so much about the blood pressure, but I'm afraid after even one drink, I may get all screwed up. Election night, however, there will be no bourbon left behind is that is one of my quadrennial events.

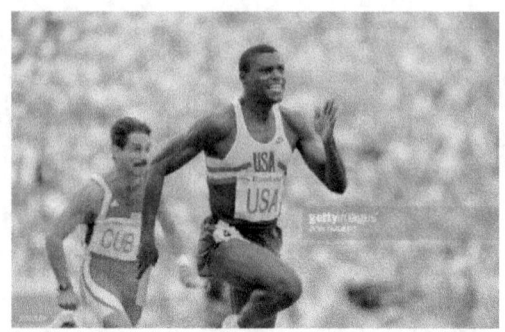

My next goal is to increase my mobility and mild use of my left hand to become more of a regular person. One of the big tests will be of course returning to work on November 14 but also preparations for my favorite day of the year, Thanksgiving. 2 Allen Place puts on a fucking show on Thanksgiving. I got my boys coming up to help, just approved by their wives today, so I'm sure this year will be extra special and I will have a lot more to be thankful for.

STEP BY STEP: THE TRIUMPH AND SUCKINESS OF INCREMENTALISM

To the misanthropic misbegotten merchants of gloom
Who look into their crystal balls and prophesied our doom:
"Let the death knell chime, its the end of time"
Let the cynics put their blinkers on and toast our decline.
Don't become demoralized by scurrilous complaint,
It's a sure sign that the old world is terminally quaint.
And tomorrow's gonna be a better day,
No matter what the siren voices say
Tomorrow's gonna be a better day,
We're going to make it that way.

To the pessimistic populists who harbor no doubt,
That everything we make our way, "to hell in a hand cart".
To the snarky set, who's sniping to get,
Anyone who puts their head above the parapet.
Don't become disheartened baby, don't be fooled,
Take it from someone who knows the glass is half full.
And tomorrow's gonna be a better day,
No matter what the siren voices say.
Tomorrow's gonna be a better day,
E're gonna make it that way. Billy Bragg

These entries are becoming somewhat shorter as we move into real time. They are no longer histories, no longer chronicles of the past, but a narrative of happenings. I appreciate all of you that have read them, have commented on Facebook or mentioned posts to me. This writing has truly been therapeutic and I hope it will help others so please share. If there's anything specific you want me to write about concerning this recovery, please let me know nyalfuentes@Comcast.net

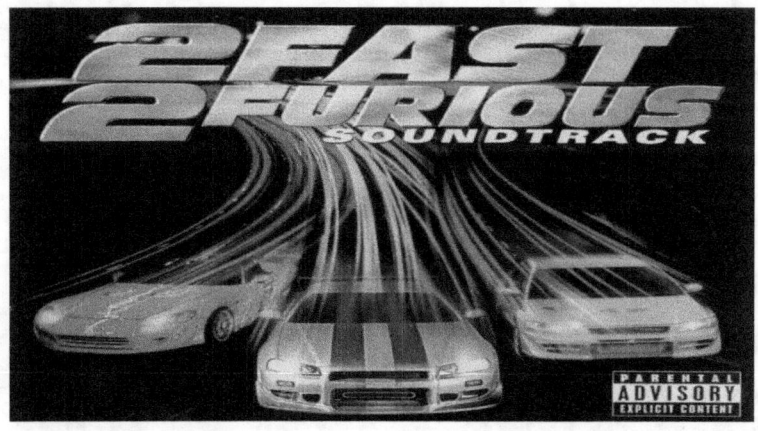

Back to the soundtrack of my life, there are certain

songwriters that stick in my head; Stevie, Paul Westerberg, Grant Hart/Bob Mould, Tupac, Chuck D, Marr/Morrissey, strummer/Jones, Chuck D and Billy Bragg above and many more. These all become part of the soundtrack that keeps you moving forward.

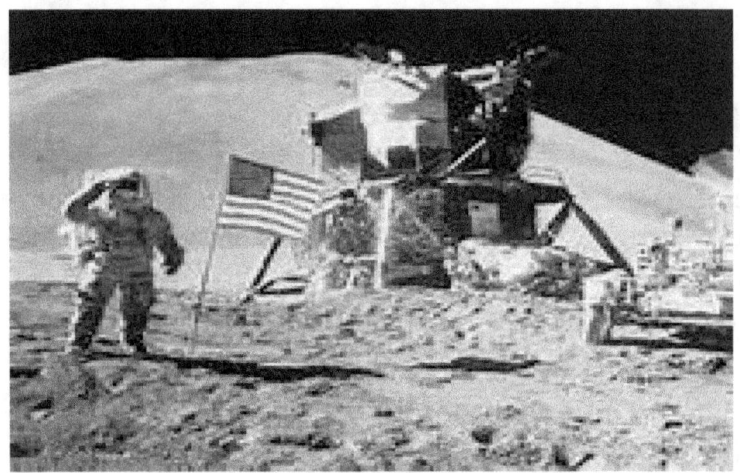

there's a moon in the sky, it's called the moon

This entry is really about incrementalism and simultaneously how important it is and how much it really sucks. Americans, and I count myself among them, most often celebrate the big event; the Fourth of July, the Super Bowl, the moon landing, V-J Day, the release of the latest Star Wars movie, etc. it's pretty easy to celebrate big events, we buy a bunch of food, yell and scream and just generally are very excited. It's much more difficult and less exciting to understand and appreciate the daily events that bring you to these big celebrations.

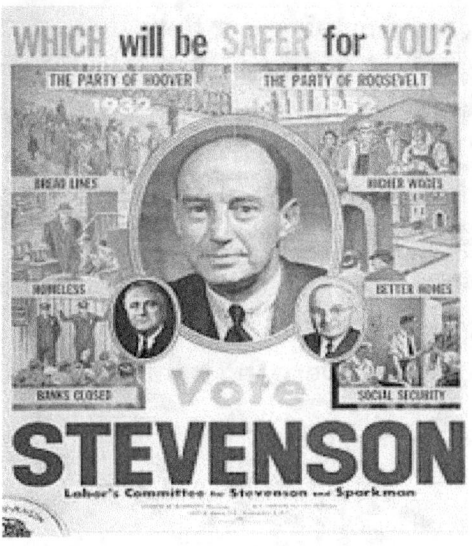

For the Fourth of July for example, I always think about this quote from Adlai Stevenson, it's one of my favorites; *"Patriotism is not a short and frenzied outburst of emotion but the tranquil and steady dedication of a lifetime."* This quote resonates with me, particularly among the flag-waving and short-term thinking of an election cycle. Patriotism like anything else takes a lot of work, it's the daily understanding of what is to be a citizen, not just voting but becoming civically engaged at every level, challenging what you think is wrong and strongly supporting what you think is right every day. All these other events had a series of day-to-day challenges as well, getting to that Super Bowl, designing the Apollo mission, all took a lot of struggle to get there.

The reason for this long introduction is that there is no real celebration of stroke recovery, there are a series of events along the way in which you work hard and have small milestones. Maybe my big celebration will be riding those 25 miles sometime next June for Tufts floating hospital, maybe it will be something else to be determined, but there is no Super Bowl or Fourth of July for recovering from a stroke. There are small things every day certainly, yesterday I did some yard work at a very slow and somewhat ineffective pace with the kids and Becky. I was probably slightly more effective than Marisol and it took me probably two hours to do poorly what I would've done effectively in probably half an hour two months ago. This incremental change is very frustrating.

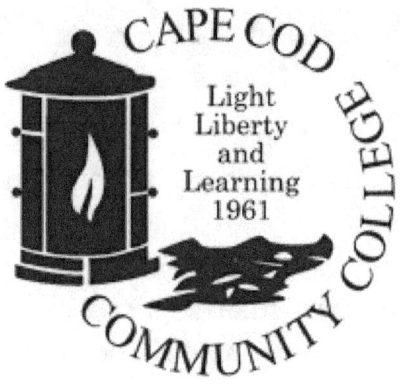

To go back to comparing this to something that is not really related is my Associates degree from Cape Cod Community College. Community college is a strange animal, and I can compare it to stroke recovery in a somewhat weird way. When you're at the college most of your friends, family and work colleagues may not be in the community college. There may be a couple, but mostly you're on your own, that's not to say that people don't support you, but they don't really understand the day-to-day of holding down a full-time job or two, commuting to school, spending time there with professors and other students just getting all your work done. In a weird way, it's the only thing I can pick that compares to what I'm doing now. Don't get me wrong, as I've often said, people support me to an incredible degree but mostly if I don't do the work, if I don't concentrate, if I don't keep a good attitude, I'm going to fail. To me community college was the same way, you cobbled together what you could, whether it be academic credits, money or time and you just get it done. If you're ever looking to hire someone and everything else is equal, hire the one with the community college degree. I work with a slew of people, perhaps a majority that went to some of the country's top colleges, Harvard and the like. I got a lot more education after community college but those work habits, that attention to detail with a lot of distractions when everything around me was chaotic have helped me to persevere. I know I digress, but that struggle has become part of my personality, my character as you would, and I'm relying on that for stroke recovery.

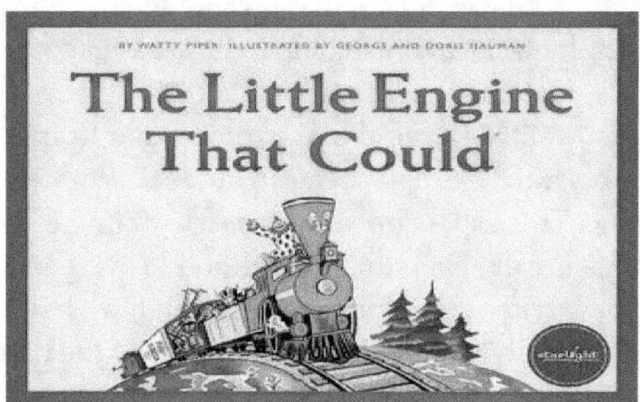

I think everyone has those moments in our lives, those moments where you overcame something, real or imagined. That becomes your fuel tank for further success. If you go back to your pre-stroke baseline you'll be frustrated daily, this morning it was a simple as finding long pants and putting them on, on what is the first real cold day of the year. Things that would take you seconds, take minutes and those minutes become hours and you don't really know where the day went.

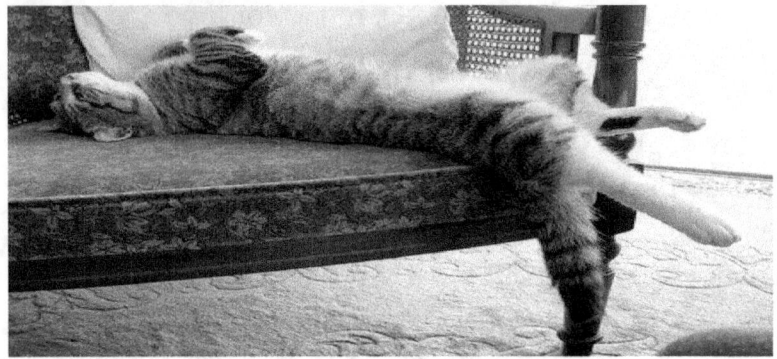

you gotta take it easy

Fatigue becomes a real issue. Some days like yesterday, I could barely stay awake, yet I really couldn't sleep. My balance was even further off due to exhaustion and I couldn't do all the exercises that I wanted to do. For those who are parents, I can only compare it to when your children are infants and at best you get 2 to 3 hours asleep, you're just walking around like a zombie and trying to care for this little, helpless creature not really knowing what to do. This exhaustion becomes frustrating as well because you really have to pay attention to every step you take and every move you make when you have had a stroke. You really want to do the exercises all the time, the PT, the OT and generally try to help around the house like you used to. But you just can't, you're too tired and it's not like lazy tired it's almost an inability to even try to will yourself into that movement, sometimes it feels physically impossible. The issue is that mobility becomes very difficult as this fatigue affects your balance. The nurses have told me that healing of the brain creates fatigue on its own. Now I've googled nothing about stroke recovery, so mostly I'm taking people at their word and it certainly feels this way. Also, the exhaustion comes from thinking about that every step, making sure that your foot is ready in the right place with the heel down first, checking around you for any possible obstacle both present and future and actually try to think about things like how I might go to get up on the curb or should I walk around and find a curb cut or how am I going to open that Tupperware container. These things that you always took for granted become what I call an adventure in daily living.

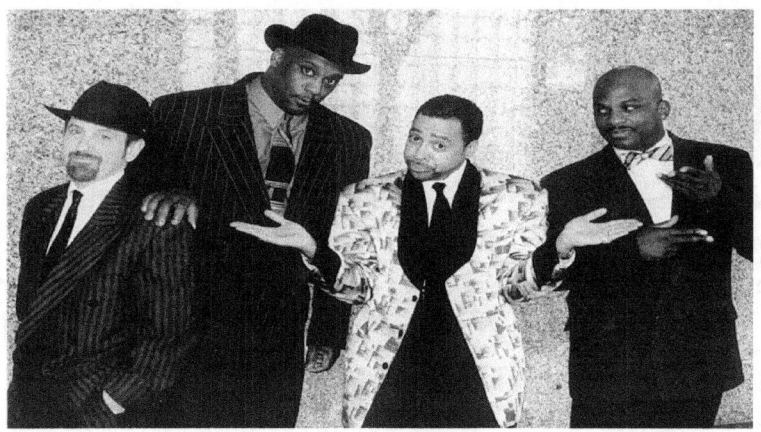

no not that time, Jerome

So, time becomes both your friend and your enemy. When you're looking at incremental change you sometimes have to see everything as a triumph, yesterday I emptied out all the dead flowers next to my patio, that may have been my major accomplishment for the day. In the past that may have been a 15-minute activity before getting on to the rest of my day, now essentially is the best part of the day. When dedicated to incrementalism you have to appreciate every one of these small benchmarks are else you'll lose your mind. In some ways that's my struggle, I want the big success, I want to play a game of basketball or ride my bike around the Lake in Wakefield. But those things can't happen for a while, until then, it's getting up and down stairs, maybe even switching legs as I walk up or trying to pull all the dead sunflowers out of my gardens, it's a short walk with my neighbor Steve to the bank and get a cup of coffee. The hardest part when you're a relatively high achiever and somewhat successful is to appreciate all the successes as a part of a bigger success at the end. My next two high-level goals at this point are to return to work in three weeks and be able to be a solid contributor and also being able to cook a large Thanksgiving dinner and have the best Thanksgiving ever (this is always our goal in the Fuentes family). Earlier I stated that most this effort is "on me". While that is mostly true having all your support along the way is incredibly important, while I tend not to seek praise for everything I do, I have to admit getting some credit along the way is pretty damn important. I appreciate being recognized for my efforts I think if you're working with a stroke patient it is important to recognize these efforts without pandering which I think can be challenging, we don't want to be treated like little kids who need encouragement for every little thing, but also want to be appreciated for efforts. It's probably a weird line to travel.

Again, I want to thank everyone for their patience, believe me this much more frustrating for me that is for you. I'm a guy who tends to be pretty self-sufficient, stubbornly does not ask for help with anything at this incrementalism, the speed at which everything is moving, really starts to make you crazy. But this is not a choice, there is no magical medical treatment, no drug, no therapy, that can make this happen any faster. You just go with it, do the work, try to smile and enjoy life. Please join me on this journey.

Frustration: the anatomy of recovery

Nothing ever happens to people like us
'Cept we miss the bus, something goes wrong again
Need a smoke, use my last fifty P.
But the machine is broke, something goes wrong again

Something goes wrong again
And again
And again, and again, again and something goes wrong again
Something goes wrong again

I turned up early in time for our date
But then you turn up late, something goes wrong again
Need a drink, go to the pub
But the bugger's shut, something goes wrong again
Buzzcocks

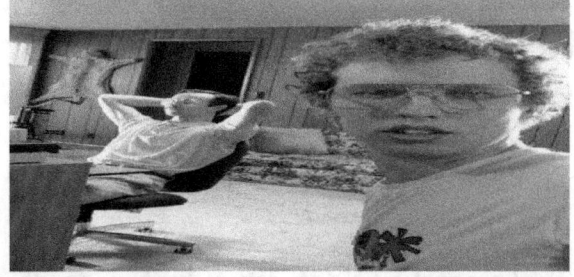

My productivity in writing has slowed down considerably. You may have noticed the chapters about incremental change are just not as exciting as the preceding events. It is difficult to tell the change from one day to another. There is a general sense of frustration as time goes along. I'm nowhere close to 100%, which always leads you to fear that you will never be hundred percent again. Granted I can do things I didn't dream of six weeks ago. I've managed to go a lot of places on my own, even taking and switching buses to get back from a doctor's appointment. I've been lucky to still have a lot of help – people from church taking me to appointments when my wife is at work and generally just being the crazily supportive people that they are. We even had a youth group come over and pick up a lot of leaves in my yard and bag them up. I'm not a super religious person. I struggle with faith every day but the people in my congregation are unbelievable, to the point that Rebecca and I are often stunned. Congregations like ours just attract positive, supportive people full of love in their hearts. We have definitely found the right place to worship. But as usual, I digress.

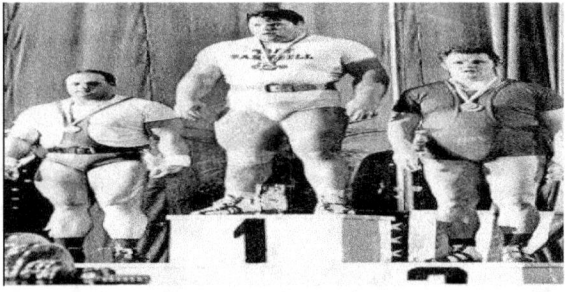

I'm in OT and PT twice a week now. It's no longer the job it was when I was in Spaulding. I don't wake up every morning and have therapy first in my agenda. I don't have to just wait to be picked up by my therapist. It just becomes another part of your routine for those couple days a week. Most of your work is around exercises at home. And, of course, your adventures in daily living. I've managed to start going back to the gym at least a couple days a week. I ride the bike and do some light weights on machines. I can't really lift over my head due to a shoulder weakness but I am definitely moving along. It's funny though to be working with a cane as you move through the weight room where people are doing feats of strength.

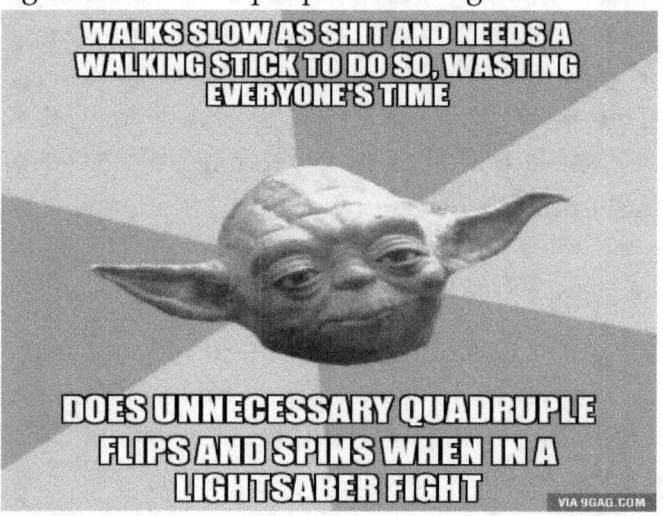

My independence has definitely grown. I can get up and down stairs on my own confidently. This week I managed to walk a half a mile to the library, check out some movies and come back another half-mile without any real struggle. Generally everything is going pretty good; if I had to guess I'm about 40%. Six weeks ago I was about 3%, not that there's any real scale of this. In the middle of the night I can grab my cane and go to the bathroom on my own if need be. For norms, I imagine you all take this for granted I certainly did.

On the other hand, I can't do fairly simple things that I always did. I could not put up a spice rack because my left hand has strength but not a lot of control to keep something level. I couldn't walk to the basement to get the drywall anchors I needed and now have to wait for someone else to help me. I managed to cook a large spread for election day, but definitely felt limited. I lacked some confidence in moving a large crockpot of beans, for instance, and generally getting heavier things out of the oven is very challenging. Even a half sheet pan of baked stuffed potatoes took concentration and effort when ordinarily I'd just grab a dry rag and toss it on top of the stove. Still the meal came out pretty good even if the election itself did not. I managed to make a gravy from roux and multitask in making a fairly large meal.

You just don't notice the difference day-to-day. When I go to my PT or OT twice a week, they seem to think I'm making progress. One example is running into our friend Joe Murphy, the plumber who is really excited to see the progress I've made. Thing is, where do you set your baseline? Is my baseline crippled Nyal, September 6 Nyal, or 23-year-old Nyal? At one point when we were at Market Basket and I was pushing the cart, I attempted to jog with the girls across the parking lot. It just seemed absurd, like I would never be able to run although I tried. I can move at a pretty good clip now and have a decent gait but when I get tired it gets sloppy.

On election day, we had a good-sized party with the food I talked about, but we are all super depressed about the outcome. In an ordinary year I would consider this to be the very bottom of my year, but I can't say that this year. To be honest it's not quite equivalent but almost. Over the past two months I feared for my future physical health and hoped that I would be able to recover and be strong as I was before – physically, emotionally and mentally. I now fear for all of us, an unqualified orangutan in charge of the strongest and greatest country on earth. I'm not one of those tolerant progressives and I'm completely intolerant of intolerance. I feel like I have to muster the strength to at least do my small part to drag my country out of the ditch that they've chosen to drive themselves into. As I've stated before it's hard to imagine not being able to protect your family, to be physically unable. Now I feel I have to do so much more which adds to the stress getting better. But this isn't a political tome so I'll just leave this here.

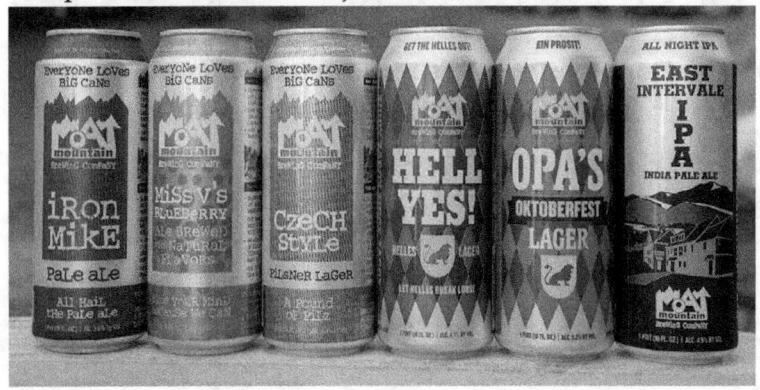

I did manage to have my first drinks on election night so maybe that's progress. I don't imagine I'll drink like I used to but, boy, from time to time it feels good to have a few drinks with your friends and just loosen up a little. There is also the realization that nonalcoholic beer sucks in comparison to the wonderful craft beers that are out there.

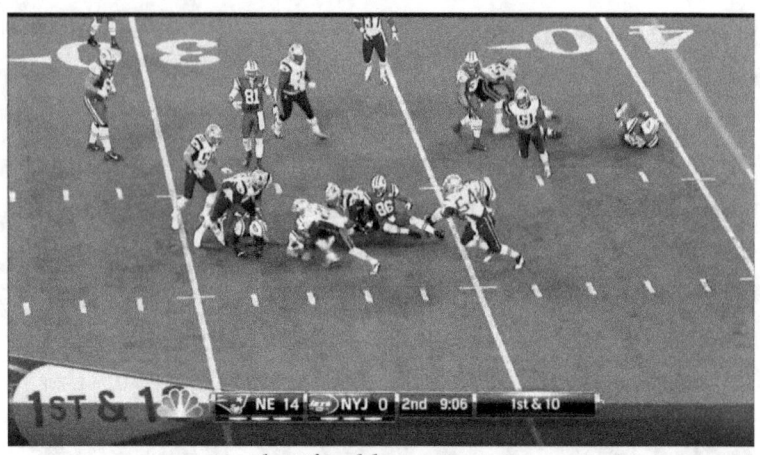
buttfumble recovery

I imagine in all recovery there is frustration. Many people such as my mom that are "in recovery," would probably say that recovery lasts a lifetime. I imagine recovering from a stroke is somewhat the same. Over time there'll be a lot of normal things returning, like not worrying about your foot placement when you get out of a chair. Elena and I went to a presentation on Tuskegee airmen the other day at Melrose high school. As it was very well attended, we ran into a lot of people we know; many of the same do-gooders we see around town. Elena and I like to do these nerdy things. Usually she is a bit tentative and will think things are boring but since we're kind of wired the same in many ways, we're just interested in everything. But at one point the stroke strikes again. I stood up funny without concentrating and fell to my knees on the carpet. I was fine but again I became a center of attention to all around me. I was that crippled guy again and not just a normal guy trying to get his learn on. As time goes on, I have to remember to not be mentally lazy about my temporary disability, to take that extra second to do things the right way.

It is hard to remember that "this too shall pass" – that someday, I may be standing in front of a chair in someone's backyard swinging a wiffleball bat, grabbing a cold beer and throwing Marisol into a bounce house all within the same 45 seconds. That I'll get a chance to be "the monster" chasing the kids around at a barbecue while ragging on Fred for saying something stupid. It's the combination of all these things, the living of life, real life where there is a lot going on at the same time that I wish to get back to.

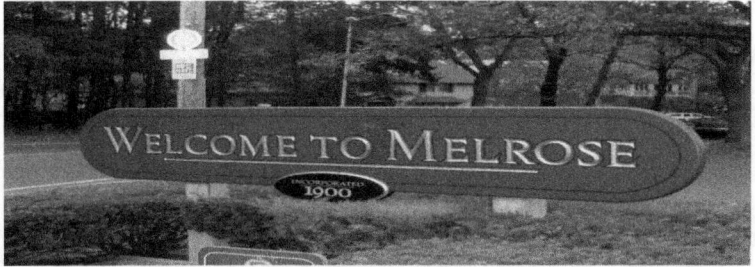

This Monday I start back at work, it's supposed be part-time but probably spend about 20 or so hours in the office and another 10 at home. Additionally, I don't have my driving privileges back yet so I'll have to concentrate on buses and rides from family and friends to get back and forth. I look forward to some of these transitions being a lot less difficult. I'm lucky to live where I do and have a walkable city and access to transportation to get me around locally. Recently I've been thinking that Melrose is probably a great city to age into. You can get access to all of your regular daily requirements, bank, crappy grocery store, post office, library, CVS, as well as about 11 pizza joints and some fine food and drink. I'm thankful for the choices we made around this lifestyle, frustrating as it is to get a great cup of coffee or some Mexican food. Outstanding seafood helps to alleviate that frustration.

Recovery can be frustrating, mostly because you can't really see it yourself. You have to judge yourself on how others see you. Well not judge per se, but mostly evaluated or given context about. I hope to have the strength to keep up the day-to-day.

Back to work

Ooooh…
 You might not ever get rich
 But let me tell you it's better than digging a ditch
 There ain't no telling who you might meet
 A moviestar or maybe even an Indian chief-Rose Royce

Humans don't mind hardship; in fact, they thrive on it; what they mind is not feeling necessary. Modern society has perfected the art of making people not feel necessary. It's time for that to end."
— **Sebastian Junger,**

Let's be clear, there are few people in the world who really enjoy their jobs, Hugh Hefner maybe, maybe some professional athletes, reality TV stars, but I'll bet even that gets tired. Most of us would probably do something else than going into an office or other workplace, going to a bunch of meetings, sitting in a cube and dealing with people all day and that's not even mentioning the phone or the commute. Everything else aside if we just got a big check every week or two, we probably could find something a lot better to do, maybe I would just grow tomatoes or learn some type of new hobby. Since I'm not a

trophy husband, I need to go out and bring home the
vegetarian bacon.

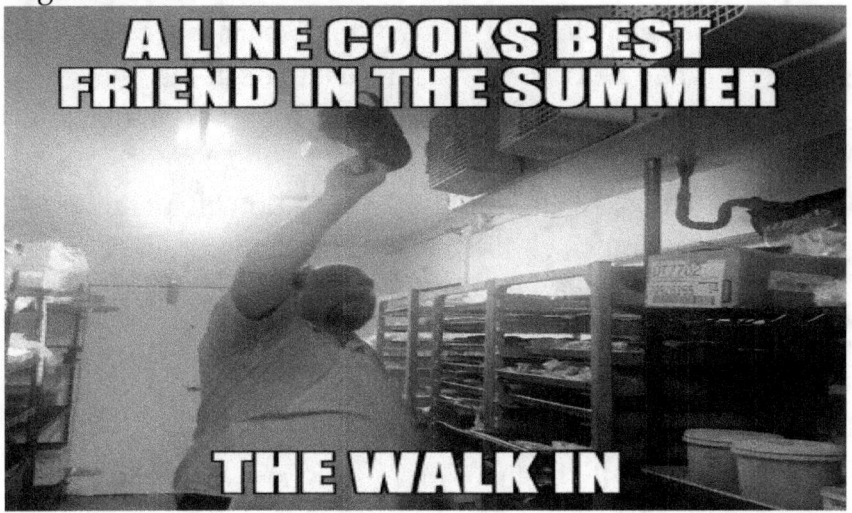

A LINE COOKS BEST FRIEND IN THE SUMMER

THE WALK IN

There is value to work, intrinsic value as well as the
obvious financial compensation we need to get by in a
capitalist society. We live in a world where some of the
hardest workers are the least compensated. Some of the
hottest, dangerous, and grueling jobs also pay the least
money. Education can alleviate a lot of those characteristics
of labor but as they say "mo money, mo problems." One of
my biggest goals was to have a career that paid well, was
fulfilling, but most of all one where taking a shower was
optional and not required when you got home. Most of my
younger life was spent in what most people would
consider crappy jobs. Growing up on the Cape in the 80s,
most kids went to work as soon as they could get a
working permit, in those days I think views of child labor
were closer to the 1910s than the 2010s. It was not unusual
for 14 and 15-year-olds to work 60 and 70 hour weeks late
into the night from the early morning in kitchens and other

places. In a lot of cases teen labor filled the spots that immigrants do today in the Cape's economy. I learned a lot of my work ethic in those kitchens and learned from both good and bad bosses what it was like to be in the workforce. I had some pretty shitty jobs and I don't look fondly back on doing stuff like fishing a dead squirrel out of a grease bucket, cleaning out the tampon bin at the Natick Marshall's, working sick, injured and often hung over and other trials and tribulations of being in the lower service economy.

Nonetheless, there is dignity in work and since I had my stroke I was really looking forward to returning to work. Again as much as a job as a job, I've always felt my work is important, it is a small part, and a very small part of improving education in the Commonwealth, of working with schools, districts, principals, teachers, counselors, and other educators to build a better system to serve our youth and families.

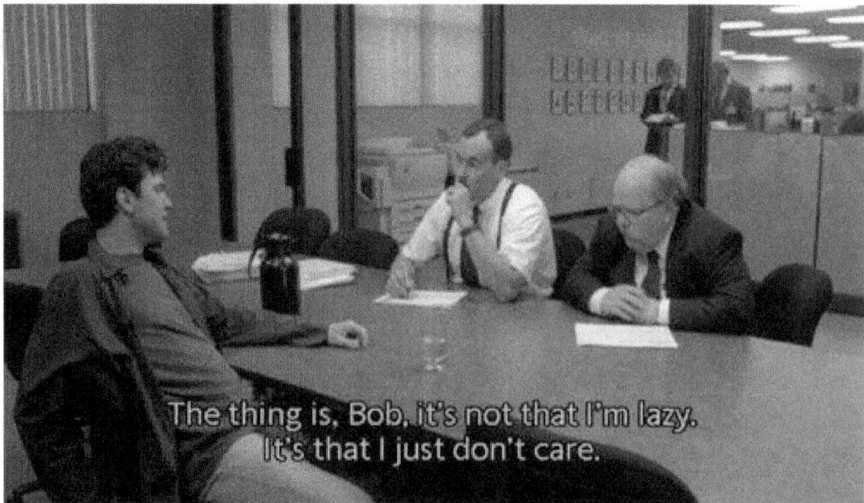

The thing is, Bob, it's not that I'm lazy.
It's that I just don't care.

After two months, it was time to go back. There would be some limitations, ordinarily my work might take me all across the state, initially and currently I'm not supposed to drive a car so that creates a limitation of actually going to schools and districts. That's not to say there's plenty of work I can do in my office and put together, in fact that is become the majority of my work in recent years. Since returning home, I've developed some independence, the ability to make lunch, go to the bathroom and everything else I took for granted before my stroke was slowly coming back. Luckily as far as getting to work and my appointments in the morning, my wife was able to drop me off at those places. Also because I live in urban area, public buses easily can ferry me from home and from my therapies and to and from my place of work in Malden.

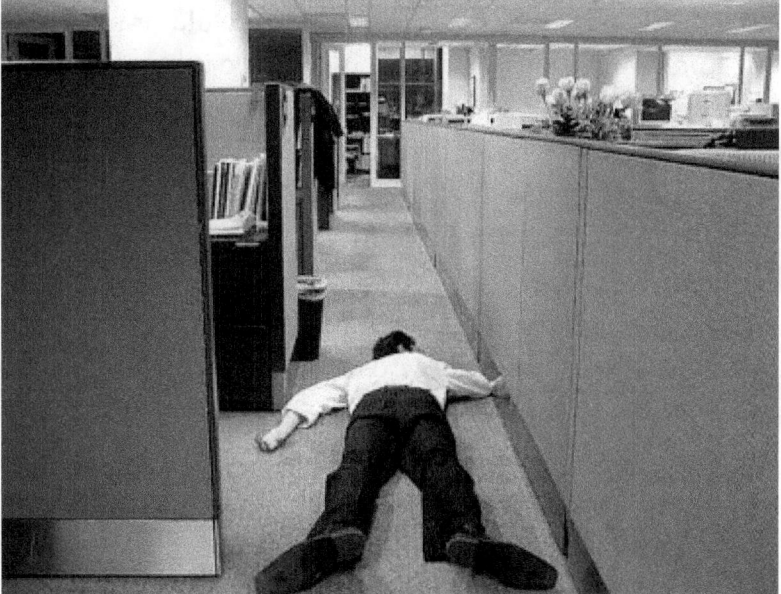

For those of you recovering from stroke or have someone recovering, outside of the mobility in my case, the biggest issue is the fatigue. As I've said before, for those who have children, it is the same exhaustion you felt when they were infants even if you're getting sleep. It's not like work is making more tired I'm just as tired, it's just the need to function in a more complex environment with a ton of different people that you may not be used to dealing with for a couple months.

Generally, people who go into education are decent folks who are do-gooders, this definitely helps in the transition. It's important for people to understand at least in my case, that cognitively I'm fine, but being so tired, makes you less likely to pick up on every detail and have the patience to participate in every conversation. I think also there is a tendency after you've had some type of brain injury for people to try to talk to you like you are a child or hold you with some pity. I mean I do feel for people it is a delicate balance, that is being compassionate, so when in doubt just ask, we are still the same person before our injury albeit perhaps with an entirely different outlook on life. I know that sounds contradictory, but in some ways although we are damaged, we are going to come out of this even better than we started maybe with a little less strength, speed and power as we play in the low post.

Newton's laws

<u>1st law</u>: *Law of inertia*
Every object continues in its state of rest, or uniform motion
in a straight line, unless acted upon by a force.

<u>2nd law</u>: *F=ma, or a=F/m*
The acceleration of a body along a direction is
  − proportional to the total force along that direction, and
  − inversely the mass of the body

<u>3rd law</u>: *Action and reaction*
For every action there is an equal an opposite reaction.

There's some stuff at work that has moved on somewhat
and you're trying to catch up on to where it moved to in
some slow-paced form of whack a mole, sometimes you
need to find out on the day that your work life froze, where
that stuff wandered off to. There is a certain Newtonian
physics to it, the issues of inertia and chaos theory collide
quickly. There is also stuff that has literally been frozen in
time, stuff that is exactly where you left it. A huge issue is
just determining what it is you do around here. Quickly I
began to realize there was lots of stuff to do in the real need
to prioritize and plan both immediate and long-term steps.
The issue of working in a large scale bureaucracy, is that
usually your work is not your own, it intersects across the
agency and across the state and there's a lot to keep in
mind with all these moving parts. I have a tendency not to
get overwhelmed, I think they call it eating the elephant.
The idea is that you're not cannot eat the elephant in one
sitting, you gotta visualize eventually finishing it, but also
breaking apart into manageable pieces.

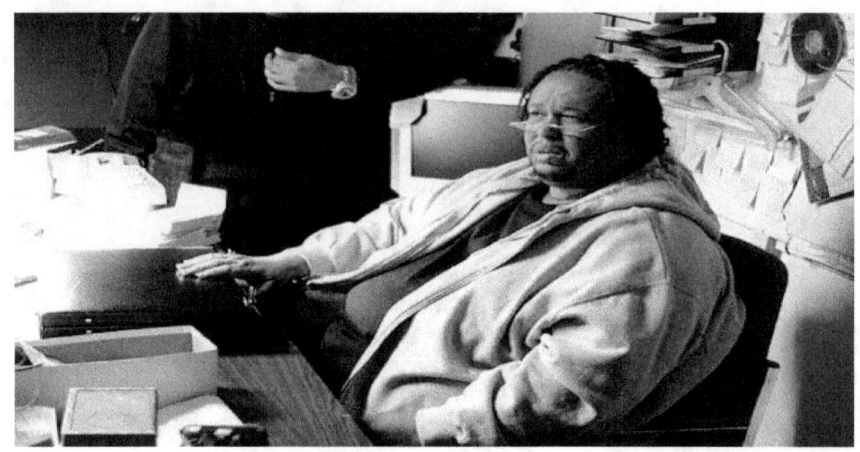
I have a proposition

I've just finished my first week, a lot of it is socialization, everyone's going to come up to you and see how you doing, and want to chat with you, that's an important part of the job. Mostly I want people to see me as the same positive, relatively happy and joking person who is still very serious about the work. I then remembered how much I actually like working with these folks, dedicated, intelligent, hard-working people with an honorable mission for the most part. While it's hard at some points to pay attention in long meetings or particularly on conference calls where I found I was hearing from the people that I really didn't want to hear from and actually forgotten about, more work acquaintances than colleagues that I found really exhausting.

And the most important thing to learn and particularly because my job isn't really physical but does require concentration is to appreciate your limitations. While inside your heart and soul you're the same person with the same internal drive and fortitude, that thunderbolt has temporarily limited your physical stamina and drive. For me, this Dragon software helped. When I took a typing test the other day at OT, I typed 18 words per minute. With the software I was able to come up to my normal typing rate and not have the frustration of moving along at a tortoise's pace in communication. I encourage everyone returning to work to swallow your pride a little bit and take advantage of any of the opportunities available to you under ADA or any other rules and regulations of your organization or agency. I've grown to appreciate all these protections and realize that most of us will take advantage of these as we age and are still important, productive members of society.

I also have to say in closing, how much I appreciate my employers my supervisor, my fellow employees and management in helping make this work. They've allowed me to adapt my schedule and be very flexible in allowing me to contribute to our collective process. Again, those returning from injury are anxious to become productive members of society as part of our rehabilitation and to give back all that has been given to us, whether my society, our coworkers or our families and friends.

Being Papa

I ought to leave enough hot water
For your morning bath, but I'd not thought
I hate to hear you talk that way
But I can't bring myself to say I'm sorry

The past is always knocking incessant
Trying to break through into the present

We have to work to keep it out
But I won't be the first to say it's over

I used to want to plant bombs at the last night of the proms
But now you'll find me with the baby, in the bathroom,
With that big shell, listening for the sound of the sea
Billy Bragg

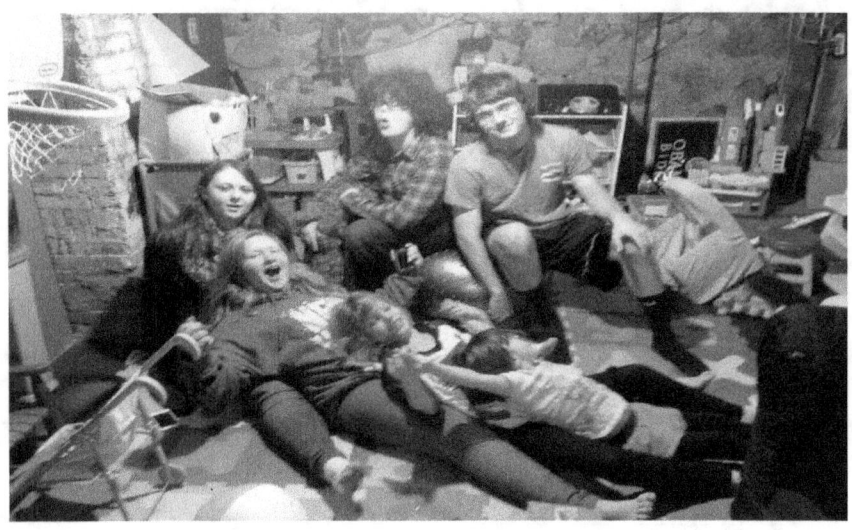

For most of my life, I was pretty content with being an uncle, with working with kids in schools and not necessarily having the day-to-day responsibility for raising a child. I could never really imagine how much my life would change once I had my kids. I was pretty good with other kids, having patience, understanding and a willingness to just yell when I needed to and not be angry all the time. Having your own kids is a complete different world. Obviously, the whole pregnancy and preparing the house was super important, but you never really know the intensity of the responsibility that one has for bringing up a decent human being. It starts in the whole birthing process and witnessing that miracle, but it really hits you, when a nurse says to you, "okay you can go home now." And you're like "really", we have no idea what we are fucking doing. It's surreal in this day of government overreach and the nanny state that perhaps the most important thing you'll ever do is unlicensed and virtually unregulated. When Elena was a day old, it was Christmas Eve and we were headed home, although the car seat was installed, we had really no idea of how to actually put this living being into said car seat and leave the hospital, yes, if you're having your first one, always practice how to do this, you'll be tired and not interested in learning new things.

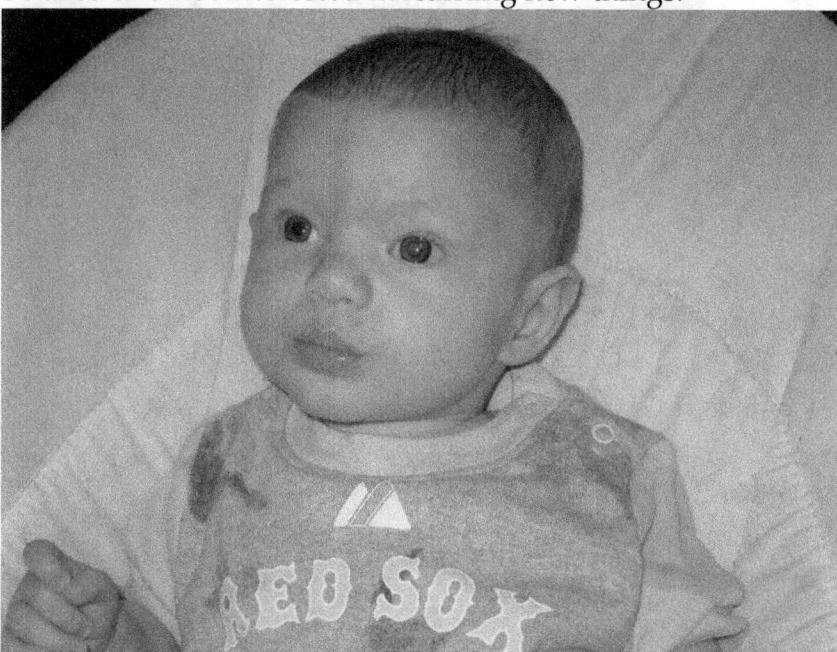

Having children was like being reborn yourself, you are an entirely different person, you're a mom or dad. The only thing I can really compare my stroke to was this feeling of becoming a parent. It was equally as exhausting albeit having the children was exciting, positive and new as opposed to depressing, dark and terrible. Nonetheless, a major part of my recovery is becoming Papa again.

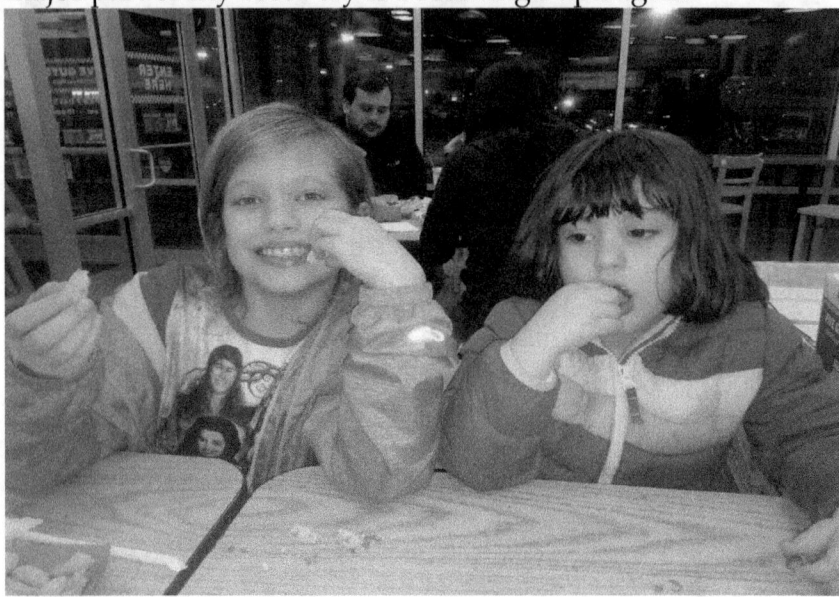

Most of you who are reading this know me and my children. For those that don't I have two interesting and active little girls who I've referred to frequently in these writings. They are absolutely different and both of them take a little bit in personality from both me and my wife. My almost 10-year-old, Elena is a super student at school, tall and pensive and is very helpful to other adults but often a pain in the ass at home, Marisol, my six-year-old is a maniac, can be loud and obnoxious and as one of my friend's states, "she's feisty" and is just a crazy ball of energy, she also behaves in school but at home is sometimes a piece of work. I think most people, both adults and children enjoy their company but I'm pretty biased.

I was a pretty active person. I spend most of my off time in the spring, summer and fall kind of futzing around the backyard and working in my gardens, I try to drive my girls out there who don't really help but I get to laugh at when they play all the games they make up in the silly things they do. My best days are these, a beer or two, podcast and music and watching my girls be silly and creative without a real care in the world.

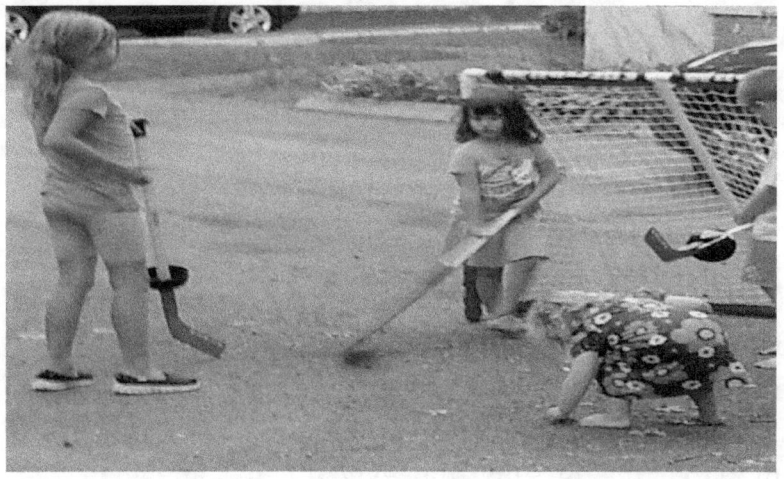

I was scared that I would lose all the fun parts of being a father and perhaps a lot of the necessary parts. I was never afraid like some people in my situation of being here to put food on the table, provide for their every need and whim or support them economically. I know that I am blessed in this fact, we are financially sound. What I was thinking more about was the affective pieces of parenting. This has not entirely gone away, doing things like taking the bikes of the shed or taking the kids on walks through the city still seem like a struggle. Teaching Marisol to ride a bike right now seems like a bit of a pipe dream. Elena took a lot of sprinting up and down Allen Place holding her handlebars before she could actually ride, physically I saw a lot of work towards. We have had a couple times in the backyard, including one special day where Marisol was raking leaves into a pile as I was leaf blowing the gardens and patio, it's days like this that mean the most to me. I need to work myself up to hikes in the Fells and trips to the science Museum and things of the like that really make me feel more full as a parent. As we speak, Rebecca is helping the girls to clean their room, as simple movements of being able to pick multiple things off the floor over a long period of time are still impossible to me. I look forward to those days where it is as automatic as it was in the past.

In the hospital, I was terrified of not being able to be whole again, slowly this is coming back, a return to work has assisted me. Going to some community events with my kids has made me feel better. Having Elena and even Marisol help me out from time to time and having them seem to treat me the same way even if I am somewhat physically slow has been an important part of the healing process. At one point I even managed to pick Marisol up and throw her on the bed and we even started do a little bit of our fighting and karate.

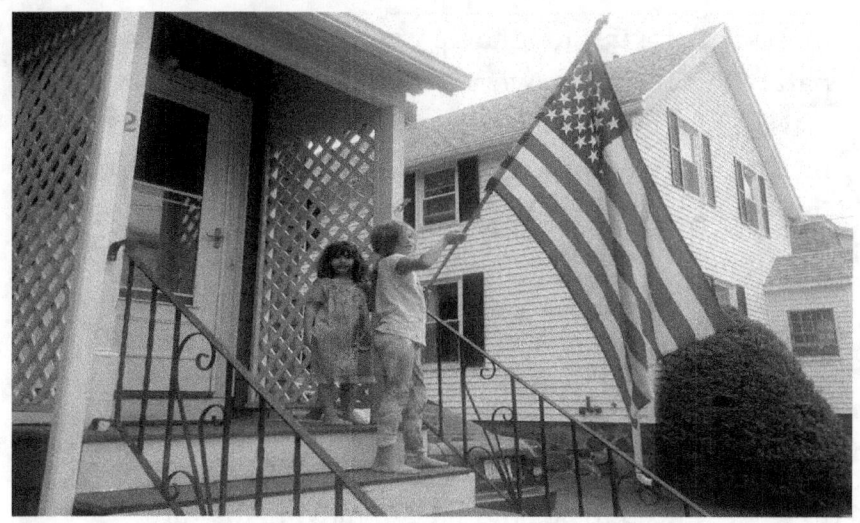

Being a parent is the hardest, most exhausting but also most fulfilling thing I've done in my life. I'm never more proud when someone else says how well my kids are doing in school, moments when they have showed compassion or empathy or helped somebody else. It is impossible to explain to someone who is not a parent how these things feel.

We are now moving in the holiday season, in fact me and Clubba go on our annual Christmas shopping trip tomorrow morning. This Thursday is my favorite day of the year, Thanksgiving is a day filled with children and adults, communing together in gratitude amongst an incredible bounty of food, drink and love. It's during this holiday season, that I hope to solidify a major piece of my recovery with my children. Some of this is physical and some of what I will struggle with, how to put the Christmas tree up, how to get the decorations out of the attic, how to organize all the dinners and do the traveling I need to do.

But with help, this too shall pass. That seems to be a major part of this whole recovery, "this too shall pass" is a consistent reminder that a lot of what is happening to me is fleeting and temporary and that I will always be "Papa" until the day I die and beyond. It is a role that I inherited through the birth of my children, but must earn through a lifetime of work. This challenge of injury and illness is a speedbump along this arc of accomplishment. Being Papa is sometimes trying to be Superman, to be all-powerful, knowing and present and able to do everything you can and are expected to for your kids. I'm still afraid I won't get to where I need to be but I'll keep moving forward.

La GuaGua: entering the world of the norms

On the bus, watch our reflection
On the bus, I can't stand no rejection
C'mon, let's make a scene
Oh, baby, don't be so mean
They're all watchin' us
Kiss me on the bus
Kiss me on the bus
If you knew how I felt now
You wouldn't act so adult now
Hurry, hurry, here comes my stop-The Replacements

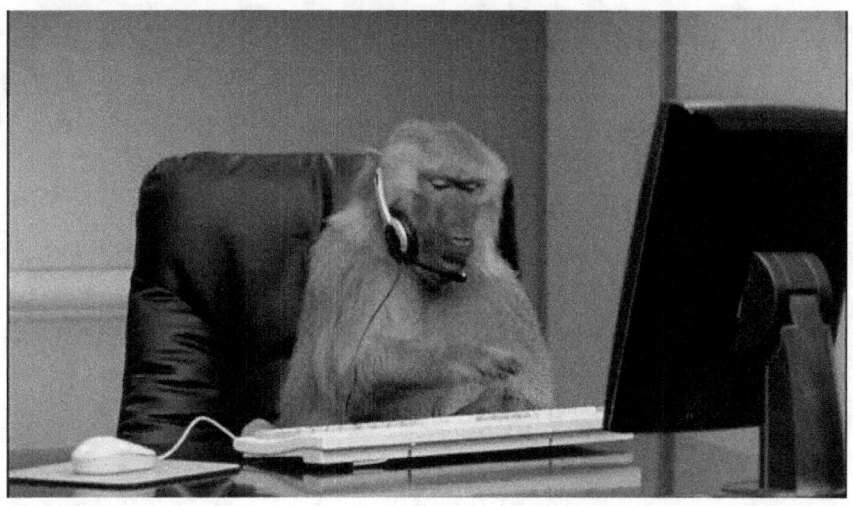

For those of you reading this on my medium.com site I now have put all of these posts in book form available on Amazon, if you're reading this in the book you already know that. I'm not trying to make any money off this but Amazon has some minimum prices. If you're local and you want one let me know and I'll get one for you. If you're interested in self-publishing createspace.com is simple easy.

This past week was December 7, Pearl Harbor Day it was also the three-month anniversary of my stroke. The stroke was a very personal version of this historical tragedy, after Pearl Harbor this country united militarily, emotionally, economically to defeat the Axis in some way, on a very micro level with no disrespect meant to what a real deadly struggle the war effort was, the day of the stroke is a day of infamy. And the recovery shows the multilevel effort and struggle to get better. Now is the time so they tell me that many stroke survivors start to get depressed, you made a lot of progress but you're not where you want to be. I'm not really depressed, but I am frustrated from time to time to just be able to do everything like I did in the past. For example, I took a typing test at OT and typed 18 words a minute so I'm sticking the Dragon for the time being. What used to be ordinary is still kinda difficult, for example I'm not driving yet and the stairs in the subway are still pretty challenging. So this is the continuing effort to go from "Crip" to "norm" in every facet of life possible. One of the things has made my life somewhat more normal is taking the bus, that's not to say that anyone who takes a bus is normal, the crosscut of life particularly in the middle of the day in the non-rush-hour times is not normal at all. It is a very strange group of folks. One of my favorite words in Spanish but may be particular to Puerto Rico is" la guagua". For some reason, this word sounds onomatopoeic, the slow rumble of the bus tires over city streets kinda makes a sound like that word. Transit apps have made bus taking much easier and you get little walks in to get some exercise. And there are crazy ass people on the bus; nose pickers, people yelling at each other, junkies, you name it. But nonetheless it is maybe more normal, I can get places without being dropped off like a little kid. Not to say I've been a big fan of normal in my life anyway. I treasure time with unusual people with strong critical thinking skills, the ordinary is often quite boring and we sometimes live in a society that treasures linear and mainstream thinking.

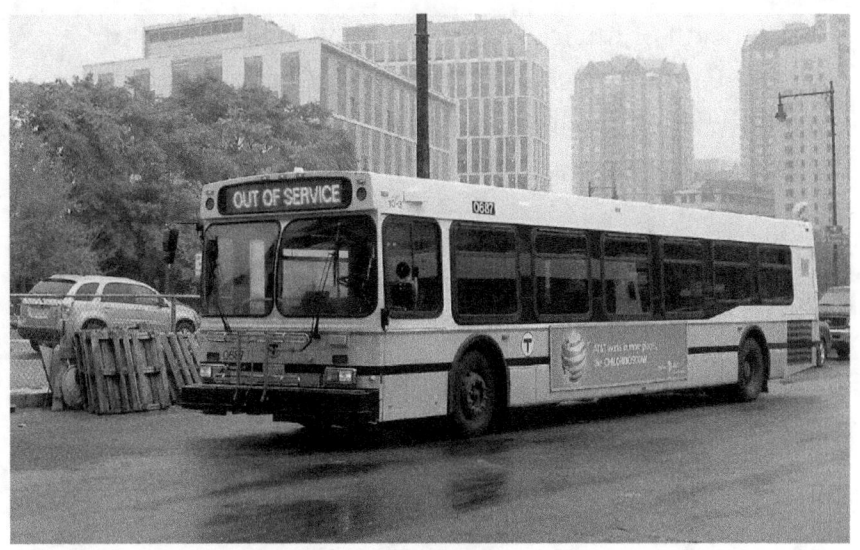

Over the past couple weeks, I've also managed to go on a couple of walks, these walks are mainly because the bus runs much more infrequently mid-day and I have no desire to wait a half an hour when I can make the walk in 45 minutes. I've managed to walk home from work three times, this ambulation commute is 2.1 miles. I'm doing it with a cane still but the cane starts it starts to not be so much as a crutch, if you would to mix my medical metaphors. With the cane at this point and as time goes on you start get used to it and becomes an extension of your body and is mainly used for curbs, negotiating holes in the ground and checking for ice. Ice and snow will be a real test, if you lived in New England for a long time you tend to learn how to walk in snow and ice, you'll see tons of people scurrying around in penguin like small steps to negotiate the weather. You know to wear appropriate footwear and to keep your feet, head, hands and private areas warm at all cost and to stay dry. One of the most difficult parts of my day due to a shoulder subluxation that was a result of muscles atrophying because of the stroke is to get my winter jacket on, again something never would've thought about in the past, you need to develop your own methods to do what you would do automatically in the past.

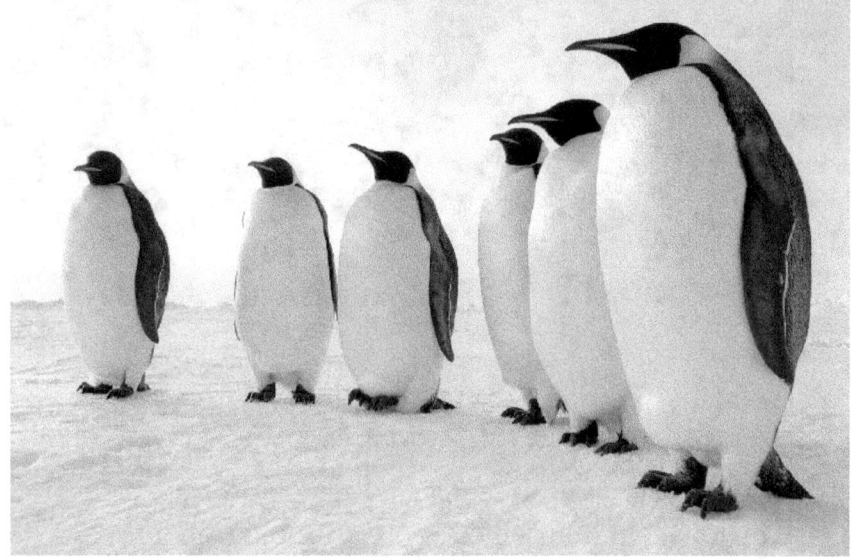

Bus stop in Malden

I'm still not quite norm status, people still come up to me and say "you're amazing", I do appreciate it and very thankful that people recognize the efforts but in some ways it feels weird. Helen Keller was amazing; I'm just trying to heal well. And I imagine you are not truly a norm until people stop saying that you look good because how often do you really tell someone they look good in normal conversation. There still will be times when people talk really slow to me or are a little bit condescending in speech or mannerisms. I think this probably is because I didn't have the cognitive issues that others who have had strokes did or maybe they've always talked to me this way and I never noticed.

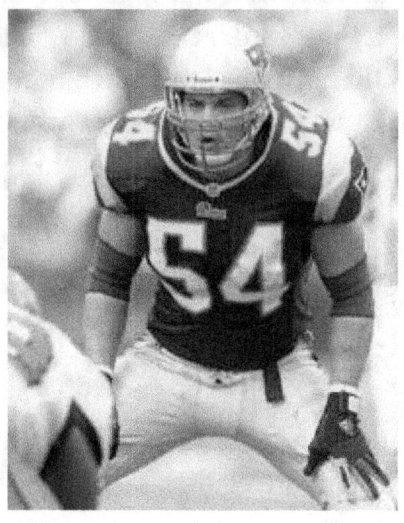

Tedy Bruschi played NFL football eight months after a stroke, if I know anything about statistics, that means I should be making my NFL debut sometime during late spring training camps because causation is correlation or that's what I've heard. As humans thankfully at least most of us don't try to compare our success to those that are unsuccessful and have failed, because that is straight loser talk. We look to those who have worked hard, played fair and done well. When it comes to recovery and rehabilitation it's the same thing. One of the things I've learned is that even though you've hit bottom, don't make it your residence, get the fuck out of there as soon as you can. Much of it is boring, just like anything that you do to get successful. Bounce up as good as you can and just try to figure it out. There've been days recently that I felt a little backslide, that I was behind the progress that I've made, really just feels that way because you think you can do more. One of the things I try to teach my girls is that if you fall down on the ground, literally stand up, dust yourself off and walk around in circle a few time. These simple things are about taking control of yourself, cleaning yourself up, and then moving to realize that the short injury you just had was probably more humiliation than actual physical punishment and that nothing is broken and that you can make it happen. I'll take small things I can control over big things I can't 99 out of 100 times. There's a lot of shit you can't control, the realization of that is a huge life victory.

Nearly up to working full-time now, including trips to Boston on the T and even a ride out to a regional meeting in Central Massachusetts with a colleague of mine. I presented in front of a group and I think those who don't know may not know anything is wrong with me other than I look like a guy is way too young to be using a cane. Last night at my friend's birthday party I walked in the restroom and the guy asked me if I blew out my knee, was pretty random but his experience with a cane was a blown knee ergo the correlation causation thing again all people with canes have blown out knees. This party was processed probably a good indication that I can interact in a barroom getting to and fro ordering shots at the bar and carry them to the table and all sorts of stuff that my therapist at Spaulding would be proud of, well perhaps getting hammered would not be on the list, but it didn't fall down.

On another occasion, so was getting frustrated with me because I was moving up the stairs so slowly on the right-hand side, I could feel the breath and their sighing at Harvard station as I slowly went step-by-step, I think after he passed me he may have seen my cane hanging out my bag and he kind of smiled at me and probably had himself in embarrassment, but actually appreciated it, people getting frustrated with me, it's a little bit more normal So in some ways I've become an undercover Crip, I've managed to in many environments become just another guy, another cog in a big machine. While truly never be normal like most people at least I can pass.

Gestation

Kicking and screaming and dragged back into a life
Kicking and screaming and dragged back into a life
Like ten pounds in a nine pound bag
Still I come back to give you something that you never had

Idiot rules, I never fight I only win
Idiot rules, idiot rules
Idiot rules, and I didn't make them
Idiot rules, I never bend, I only break them- Anthrax

I haven't written since before Xmas. Six months, so much has happened, yet so much remains the same.So a quick update. I put all the previous entries into my short book, much of which are dark, forbidding memories to me. It's hard to think of some of those days, and praying of course that this does not strike me down again, because your likeliness of having another stroke after one is much higher. I'm not sure I could do it again, this road has been so terrible albeit filled with people who made heroic efforts to make it better.

It's been nine months since my brain tried to kill me. Usually in my life it was the crazy part of my brain that tried to kill me, competing in stupid contests of drinks, drugs and physical activity. 9 months is about the approximate time of human gestation, so I imagine in some senses this is my rebirth, I have an opportunity to be physically and emotionally born again.

I can do a ton of stuff I couldn't even imagine I could do previously, I jogged a mile a couple of times albeit in about 13 minutes plus, I've ridden a bike around the block a few times, used power tools and built some sturdy patio furniture, gone back to working full time plus, resumed most of my civic activities, planted my gardens, and most of all regained the ability to drive, which is incredibly liberating. No longer slave to the well organized and managed transit system around the Boston area with its well-groomed and well-behaved riders. Free to go to stores, pick up the kids, drive to and for work without having to ask anyone for help. Getting my physical mobility back was essential but being able to motor about is great, a drive to DC and back was my final exam. Below are a couple of updates about my residual struggles, partly because it is my right to complain, but to talk to other strokies.

Fatigue

It's still hard, I'm so incredibly tired all the time, stroke fatigue is real. Now at some points as I turn 50 in a couple of weeks it's hard to tell if this was just a middle-aged thing. Pre-stroke, I was able to work in the yard for 10 hours in the sun, now I struggle to work for even a short time without sitting down for a few minutes. The fatigue is beyond physical, it is mental and emotional, an almost inescapable beast. Good night's sleep, bad night's sleep not much different, albeit some days are better than others. It's often hard to keep your patience at some points and my temper can be rather short and with two young children and a job with a ton of internal and external customers my self-control can sometimes be on edge. There are points that I just like to space out and watch movies and play on social media, it is entertaining and not exhausting. I've read a bit about stroke fatigue and talked to docs, therapists, etc., and the answer seems to be, "we're just not sure". Thanks, doc, I'll just go ask Markie then.

Physical "Retardation"

Ordinarily I get around pretty well, for those of you who have followed my story, mobility has been one of my main concerns. It is a strange thing not to be able to move parts of your body, when you consciously try to move a body part and it just stays there. One of the scariest things that ever happened to me. Once I knew I was not going to die (that night that is, I'm not immortal), the fear of not being able to move was just terrifying. I thought there was a chance I'd never walk "normally" again, never be able to run around with my kids, garden, walk around the city and may even have to sell my house and move somewhere that was handicapped accessible, in other words for all that I worked my whole life to be destroyed. Luckily, and with some work on me and my therapists part I was walking pretty quickly and had an opportunity to walk into my daughter's sixth bday party.

Nine months after the incident, I'm still a little limited, my left foot placement isn't perfect and even being a centimeter off is somewhat challenging at some points. Most of the time I walk unaided but still have the cane around for when I'm tired, going on long walks, or if I'm having a couple of drinks. I've done some pretty long sojourns; for our annual Patriots Day walkabout I did our usual route, luckily Clubber was along so I was not the slowest cripple there and we managed to do a lot of walking around Gettysburg and DC so that has ceased to really be an obstacle. Downstairs are still kinda slow and I try to be sure there is a railing just in case.

One of the strangest things is a virtual inability to jump off of two feet, just little hops and still a little unsure of landing on the left foot. Also climbing is a bit uncertain, even stepping up to my raised beds are face with a bit of trepidation. I would like one of my next goals to be a hike, something I haven't really had the guts to try yet.

For several months, I also had what was called a shoulder subluxation. A subluxation is a dislocation of a joint. For a stroke survivor it is just insult to injury. Apparently small muscles around my shoulder joint atrophied to a point where the ball separated slightly, (about half an inch) from the rest of the joint, this became about three months of occupational therapy including electrical stimulation at home and hours of boring exercises to fix it. I asked my OT, what would they do if I was Tom Brady, she said the same thing, but shoot you up with painkillers, get you back in there and suffer irreparable damage. You soon realize that whoever you are, you are mortal, you are flesh and bone and time and work is all you really got going for you. It took months to just let me get my arm over my head and slowly that functionality is coming back, my next goal which I haven't really worked on, is to swim. I'm not a big swimming fan but it always came natural to me, I never understood people who can't swim, but there I was not being able to swim, not that I would drown, but I could only propel myself across the pool in a modified dog paddle.

The Plateau

Rehabilitation is exhausting. Those first few months were hard work but almost daily you felt a little bit of progress, being able to move a toe, being able to touch your fingers together, take a shower, go pee standing up, walking, shuffle jogging, stairs, all were enormous, visible and measurable metrics. The documentary later gets more complicated, the day to day or even weekly or monthly progress is not observable and a certain frustration develops. I admit I have got really lazy, some of it is due to fatigue and a lot due to the fact that I can kind of get by with what I have. You start to eat poorly, drink and put the weight back on you lost due to your lack of appetite in the hospital. Exercise when mixed with all the daily busyness of life begins to become ignored. I feel the need to break through/beyond this plateau and I'm struggling to get it going. This is what I'm calling rehab 2.0 and has a lot of general fitness goals. I'm hoping just writing about it here will get me started.

Dude, are you mental?

I had a conversation with my friend Jane the other day about depression. I don't suffer from depression. As my tio Miguel said in the hospital, "I don't have time for depression". As I said to Jane, I don't want to compare the way I feel, which I think is controllable with people who really suffer from depression. I don't want to confuse the times in which I am anxious or uptight with those who truly suffer from anxiety. Most of my mental health issues are self-inflicted, I have a terrible sin of feeling sorry for myself and afraid when I actually have so much. I have a lot of fear of this happening again and wonder, in fact doubt whether I'd have the physical, mental, emotional and spiritual strength to make it back again. I wonder if I would just bust that cyanide cap in my back molar and make it all go away. I often wonder if I can out-think, out pray, out reflect any of my mental health picadilloes. But as a wise man should have said, you can't outrun yourself. I'm blessed with a strong support network and never have really felt i could benefit from a mental health professional. I know what they are going to say and know what they are going to do, and I'll say anything just to get out of that room with them. My positive attitude I believe has brought me far. I'm actually going to try to start volunteering at Spaulding as a peer visitor, my first training session is next week. I also have decided to start going to the support group there. I've never been a fan of support groups, feels like you are surrendering, but I'm hoping the combination of the two will bring me a little more light. I joined a Facebook group of survivors and it's mixed, the positive stuff is great but there are people and I shouldn't say this because some people are just so damaged, but some are really just insufferable, just like real life normal people.

So that's the quick update, love to hear back from folks. Also for those of you that are interested, I'm likely putting together a short fundraising bike ride for Spaulding the second week of September. Haven't really done much biking, but yet another goal.

Return to Charlestown

Wrote this over a month ago, forgot to post, finished it up today. (Aug. 3, 2017)

I pretty much have decided to try to become a peer visitor at Spaulding Rehab. There is part of me that never wants to go into that building, the first time I entered it I was on my back and somewhat unceremoniously dumped into a bed for a four week stay. It's really difficult to explain how long that is to be in a hospital, although I know a lot of people have much longer stays. The idea of four football Sundays going through, an entire month of being basically tethered either to a bed, a chair on wheels and maybe if you're lucky a little time in the therapy gym. But it's not about the building, it's about the people. There are people there who saved my life. Not meaning I was going to die but keeping me from just wanting to die which is probably more important.

I had talked to Leah who was my "recreational therapist" when I was inside. An RT basically in layman's terms focuses on rehab type stuff that is more entertaining than the tortuous but necessary exercises for healing. Leah got me back on the bike albeit recumbent and we would play games and things of that nature to work on movement. She had me come in for an interview to be a peer visitor. A peer visitor is ordinarily a stroke survivor (by the way a stroke victim is someone who dies from the episode, you'll never meet a stroke victim, we are all survivors) who visits folks who have recently had strokes and are still hospitalized. The idea is that even the most highly trained professionals in neurotherapies really have no idea how it is to actually try to function after a stroke and folks that have had strokes can really help to explain the insides and outs of what's going on. Things like getting over the humiliation of the bathroom and other hygiene stuff and the real emotional ups and downs that we have.

That being said no stroke is the same, besides the actual differences in strokes, they affect our brains, bodies and souls in entirely different ways. For people like me, relatively young, with no other health morbidities, even though my stroke was pretty serious and involved almost total paralysis on one side, my recovery has been really strong. Certainly not where I want to be and I hope to push past this plateau as I mention earlier, but I have a functional life that early on, most stroke survivors could only dream of.

On Tuesday, I drove into the parking garage of Spaulding. I always find it hard to conceive of how many people made that trip to visit me that fall and made this walk and wonder what they were thinking on the way to visit. I think of my wife coming at least once a day, if not twice and the wear and tear on her life. In some ways, as much as I'm afraid of going back in the way I originally went in, I do feel like somewhat of a conquering hero upon my return. I think of how I'd struggle to roll the chair down the hall with one good arm and one good leg. I ran into all of my three main therapists, Molly, Erica and Hannah and was greeted with the most electric of smiles and firm embraces. "You look so great" is something you commonly hear at this point, as I imagine it's the shirt and tie and uprightness compared to the two black eyes, old t-shirt, and ripped shorts not so long ago. I really had imagined myself kinda dancing in and I had made sure NOT to bring the security blanket of my cane with me, unfortunately a few days before I had a street sprint with my daughters and her friend a few days before and had sprained my ankle so my deep tango turned into a slow foxtrot to impress.

I've talked a little about Jill the nurse and I have a tendency to repeat myself, but she was the night nurse, she was the one who was the last to see me as I tried to force myself into a sleep at night, often trying to keep from sobbing into a pillow, came in and made sure I had my night meds and tucked me in at night. It's incredible to think now, but I was incapable of taking off my socks and pulling a sheet over myself. I hadn't seen her in a while and I starting crying like a baby when I hugged her and she started crying as well. These are people I will remember the rest of my life.

Still haven't done my peer visitor training, but going to try to get through a fundraising bike ride first.

Holy F#ck, I'm Tired

Sing me to sleep
Sing me to sleep

I'm tired and I
I want to go to bed
Sing me to sleep
Sing me to sleep
And then leave me alone
Don't try to wake me in the morning
Cause I will be gone- Morrissey/Marr

I realize the song above is about suicide and I am not suicidal, I had a couple tough days right at the beginning, but that wasn't me, those were demons that came in with the blockage in my brain to infect my soul inasmuch as it did for my body. These pages serve many purposes for me, 1. For me to remember my journey and share it with family and friends 2. To provide information and maybe even inspiration at time for others who have been afflicted by stroke or other traumatic brain injuries 3. to just story tell and write, which is something that brings me joy and therapy even among the madness of teetering on the edge of death and being crippled. I also think just about everything is funny, even the darkest of things has a humorous edge, I mean the fact I was almost killed by a tiny clot in my brain with all the stupid shit I've done in my life, how can one not find humor in that.

People have different theories and points of view about their lives and recovery. Many are very private, only letting those that are closest to them "in". I respect that and probably should be more like that, but it's not me, I like to "live out loud", everyone for the most part can be in my business of recovery and I really have no fear about sharing anything, if you've read along in this entire blog, you've seen a lot about mental and physical health and my comings and goings over the past 11 months. I try not to put too many people out there, I'm certain that some of those even close to me would rather I shut up at times, but it's important for me to recover with some bombast. That and now that I've turned 50, I really don't give a fuck. As long as it doesn't get me fired or have my wife leave me, I'm waving that freaked up flag.

I really entered this entry (I hate people who write like that) with the thought of writing about fatigue. Then I really wanted to write about mental health. I'll save the looney tunes episode for the next blog and focus on fatigue for now. Fatigue sucks, every article you read about fatigue will talk about sleep hygiene, don't read in bed, don't watch TV in bed, etc. but that's not what stroke fatigue is all about. If you're a parent; think back to when your children were infants, you know, walking around in a fog, trying to catch a quick nap at a stop light, pouring orange juice in your coffee kind of tired. Now imagine being that tired nearly all the time with sleep really not solving the issue, that's what fatigue is all about for someone with a traumatic brain injury even months and months after the incident.

There are very few times when I'm not tired, but also I'm not sleepy, it's like having an itch in the center of you back that you can't scratch. Strangely sometimes I'll wake up at 4 or 4:30 in the morning and not be able to get back to sleep. Luckily, I'm usually able to fight through it, get through my 8 or 9 hour work day without biting anyone's head off and on occasion go to the gym or do some yard work. We managed to have a bit of a social life, but late nights are pretty rare and most of my energy outside of work is spent keeping up with my gardens (keeping my sanity) and children (losing the same). There are few things I'd rather do than garden and keep up my little refuge that I call my yard, it looks pretty good but from time to time, this joy just becomes a Sisyphean obligation as weeds start to overcome my energy and desire.

There are so many things I want to do that I just can't get to, much of my time outside of my obligations is watching a movie or the Sox, playing on social media or the internet and just relaxing in a chair, the things I know I should do; read more books, beat Elena at chess, beat Marisol, do more rehab and gym work just seem far away after knocking out the work day and maybe shopping or making supper. On occasion a basket of laundry will seem like Everest, there are bad days and good days, on good days I can build a book shelf or weed for hours listening to podcasts, other times I just sit and stare into space, as if I'm searching for some mythical body that will force out the fog.

There are some that think I'm just not paying attention at work or something, like an aging basketball player from time to time I'm relying more on wisdom and experience than whatever the equivalent is of athleticism in the land of educational policy and bureaucracy. Trying to be a wily veteran instead of jumping out of the gym. I can usually keep it together pretty well, but probably rely on others more than I used to and definitely pick my spots. At times, I do wonder how much is stroke fatigue and how much is just aging. Does everyone feel like this? Will I ever know the difference? I do wonder about the impact on those around me, both at work and in my home life and wonder if they wonder if I will ever be "normal" (well for me) again. Or maybe this is the new normal and that's OK.

I know there are many that are worse off than me, that would sacrifice everything for my abilities and capacities. Many after strokes cannot work and must collect disability to get by. I'm still able to work at a high-income job and be moderately successful at it. To enjoy most of the blessings of life. Fatigue can be crippling, you can fight through some of it, but not all.

Every Day is a Gift

Move — move — I've got the gift of life
Can't you see it in the twinkle of my eye
I can't stand up and I can't sit down
I gotta keep movin' — I gotta keep movin'
All the time that gets wasted hating
Why don't you move together and make your heart feel better.

Paul Weller

There are many days that are a struggle, for everyone not just for survivors of brain injury. We all have shitty days, we all have good days, but to paraphrase the Wire, most days are 40-degree days, nobody remembers a 40-degree day. Most days are not very memorable, we go about our business devoid of any real highs or lows.

Last week was our annual trip to Storyland and Santa's Village, it was year six and is really a highlight of the year for our kids because we ain't the traveling types. I was a little nervous, I'm pretty mobile now and my balance is pretty good but there are a series of things that you don't do everyday and really can't practice. Getting in and out of a log flume is something that is not really covered in therapies, particularly after walking around all day and there are assorted other challenges in rides. At this point 11 and a half months out, a lot of the physical challenges beyond the fatigue are pretty nuanced, an occasional foot drag, a little off balance from time to time, but otherwise pretty good to go at moderate speeds.

As we were walking around Santa's Village, a cool place albeit weird to hear Xmas music in mid-August, I ran into a gentleman slightly older than me with the telltale ankle foot brace (known as an AFO among us cool kids) of a stroke survivor. The intent of this orthotic is to prevent the foot drop and dragging off the foot. I lost mine early (mine had cats on it for you loyal readers) as I actually found it somewhat cumbersome, particularly getting on and off buses and the like, where you really wanted to have a good feel for where you are stepping.

I walked up to the guy and said "stroke"? He said, "yes" and I explained that I was about a year out, I think if you see me, and don't know, you may not realize I had a stroke, the "funny, you don't look like you had a stroke" replacing the "funny, you don't look Puerto Rican" of most of my life. As if any identity is supposed to be worn on your sleeve. We chatted for a while and he was about five years out, which of course again makes me thank God (and everyone He has given me) for the progress that I have made. After we finished talking, I sort of apologized for walking up and talking to him and he said that it was great to talk to other survivors. And then he said "Every day is a gift." I think he may have been there with young grandchildren and I ran into him and we smiled at each other several times during the day. It was the sharing of two survivors, an inside joke that both of us shared, of cheating death and disability and being able to enjoy the blessings of life.

It is hard to think of every day as a gift. Even on my 40-degree days, I have frustrations, often with others and often with myself. The mundane can sometimes be exhausting and general human orneriness can drive one to tears. The focus of some of these next entries are really around mental health. Mental health is a continuous battle for survivors, and similar to my contact with my stroke brother in Santa's Village I have found a camaraderie with others that are not elderly and have had health scares. I have a couple of friends who are cancer survivors. They have become my sisters. We have totally different experiences. Cancer is a real fucking bitch, just a terrifying monster, but to see these women stand up to that dragon is awe inspiring, the fact that they can maintain a positive attitude while still fighting brings us all strength. I can't compare myself to a cancer survivor, I had one event where my brain tried to kill me, they have their very cells turning against them. Nonetheless, they are my people. A former student of mine, who has become a good friend in her adulthood, who is much more private than I am had a stroke when she was in her early 30's, followed by some other health issues. She continues to reign strong, showing support for herself, her family and her community in a way that you would never realize she had a life-threatening episode. A long conversation I recently had with her helped me to figure out a bunch of things in my head. Another colleague and friend survived an aneurysm, she continues to work hard in her recovery, overcoming health struggles with a positive attitude. I even have a little (probably one way) camaraderie with a young daughter of friends who is a cancer survivor, her strength is empowering.

Speaking just for myself, recovery is frustrating, you want the old you back. The person who could jump out of bed, seize the day, get shit done and just come back for more. You struggle to think if that person will ever come back or if that person is gone forever. But most of all you are terrified, as much as I'd love to be the person that I was 12 months ago, my greatest fear, one that sometimes brings me to the brink of tears is being that person that I was 11 months ago.

I made the mistake, as someone who is deeply involved in data and analytics of looking at 1 and 5 year stroke survival rates about a month ago. They are abysmal, even for people under 50 with strokes. As Han Solo would say, "don't tell me the odds." Sometimes C-3PO is just kind of a dick, and you gotta go with what you think is best. Attitude is an enormous part of recovery, you could tell the people in the rehab who were really going to struggle, they had surrendered to the beast, which frankly is the easiest thing to do.

I'm not a "going to counseling type of guy", it works for a lot of people, but to be honest, I'd pretty much say anything just for the appointment to end, my experiences with psychologists in the hospital were like this and I would have as soon just made shit up than have to spend another 5 minutes talking to someone I didn't know about what was going on in my head. I think there are a number, maybe even a majority of people who get value out of this and good on them. Just not my thing, I don't need any brain readers trespassing in my mind, I'll stick to my friends and other "survivors" I did draw value from faith and my visits from Reverend Dominic but in some ways, my soul is a different part of my being.

So, as we walk through our days, I think it is always important to think, that everyone we interact with, everyone we see is fighting some type of battle, sometimes it is just a slow struggle but often it is all out war. In some ways, we are all survivors.

The Future is Unwritten

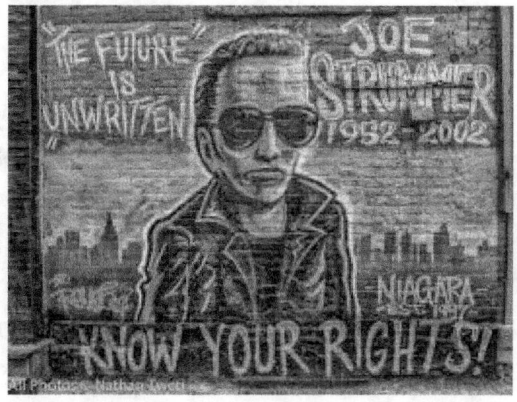

I can tell you all I know, the where to go, the what to do
You can try to run but you can't hide from what's inside of you

Any major dude with half a heart surely will tell you my friend
Any minor world that breaks apart falls together again
When the demon is at your door
In the morning it won't be there no more
Any major dude will tell you- Becker and Fagan

Before I continue with the psychological mess that is me (and humans in general) I just wanted to let you know a little about how these chapters are written. I usually sit and watch a baseball game or movie and just hammer along for a while. Today (Labor Day), I'm sitting at the table in the backyard with a Guinness listening to Steely Dan on a beautiful day overlooking my tomatoes, that have seen better days. When I wasn't working and even when I was working but pretty much immobile, it was easier to be more prolific. Now I do find it therapeutic to write, but I just don't get enough time. I also now type everything, as opposed to my earlier speech to text. Everything really is in draft form, other than what I put together for the book which an "old" family friend read for me, I just roll with it. Sometimes I'll look back at my shitty grammar or my "there" and "their" and get pretty annoyed with myself, after all most of my job is writing for professional audiences. I tend to be pretty exhibitionist in my writing, and especially when I'm talking about my own psyche and mental "stability", the conversation can be difficult. I sometimes wonder what things would look like with an editor. Because I am in the week of my one year anniversary, I'm hoping to do a couple of posts.

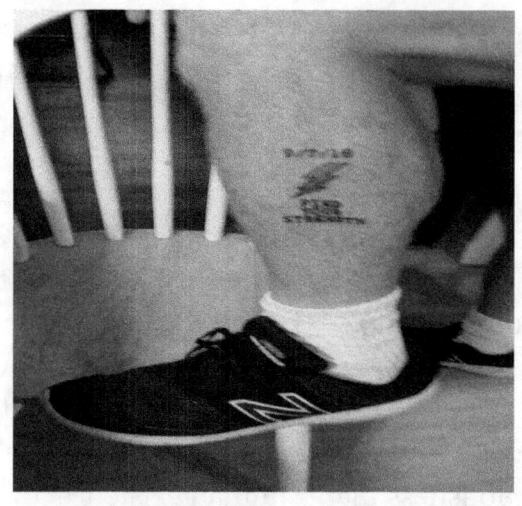

On September 7, 2016 I had an ischemic stroke, I don't
need to repeat the story in any depth here of that day, if
you have interest, the very beginning of this story goes
into a ton of detail about those first insane moments of this
journey. As a student of history, I know the importance of
knowing the past and how it provides a foundation for the
present and future. That all existence is built on previous
existence and a series of events and decision points bring
us to where we are today. I have no belief that there is
some principal architect of all of these events or any
preordained conclusion, as Joe Strummer would say, "the
future is unwritten." (He may have stole that but most of
my philosophical underpinnings are from punk rock and
rap, so what the hell do I know) There is danger in the
past, our own sometimes challenged memories and
interpretations as well as the existential regret that we
have for our own personal transgressions. The danger
exists whether we are trying to go back to an ex-, relive our
childhood, overly revere or criticize our parents and
families, or just plain trying to "make America great
again". It is important (speaking for myself and that's what

I do here) to realize that for many of us, we tend to cherry pick from our pasts, and maybe not realize that things have never been better.

One of the things I really learned growing up is the ability to survive and often thrive in chaos. There were a number of things that I screwed up but I always seemed to bounce off the bottom and do OK. I think the things that have benefited me the most include: being in on my own joke, having a pretty ridiculous work ethic when needed, my deep bench of friends and family and just a general sense of the ridiculousness that is human existence. I wonder if I had had a type A personality if this type of recovery would have been possible. Certainly someone with that type of personality would have thrilled the therapists, never have skipped the at home exercises, etc, but there really is much more to recovery, it is truly the most fucked up thing I have ever been a part of. I think spending much of my life as kind of a loser really prepared me for what I was going to go through over the past year. The sometimes loneliness and inability to get out of my own way were frighteningly familiar to me, albeit this time out of my control and this time with a strong probability of being overcome. I wonder what recovery looks like for someone that has never really faced abject failure and loserdom. If you've been to the bottom, you kind of know what it looks like and hopefully know how to get out of there. As I have said to some, eventually everyone hits bottom, the key is not wanting to stay there.

The thing is, as I sit here having this beer and typing, I'm pretty much thankfully in the same place I was last year. I read a study that said the one-year survival rate for ischemic strokes is 60% so I passed that test. I have also heard more anecdotally that most of the physical recovery happens in that first year (if not the first few months). I still feel like I got a long way to go, and in fact will test it with a 20 or so mile bike ride next week. Mostly survival as I still gotta a lot of shit to do. We are all terrified about our own mortality and me even more so I think. My entire life, I've had this existential depression and even though I lead a pretty good life as a dad, friend, husband, brother, uncle, public servant, church deacon, etc., wonder what the hell I'm doing. Flirting with the grim reaper can do that to you.

In my later adult life, I have really become disgusted with negativity and mean people. We all have our moments, there are times when I'm probably the most miserable son of a bitch to deal with. That being said there is a wide gap between being Pollyanna and being positively pragmatic. I was always impressed by the positivity of nurses; these folks had the pragmatic skills to keep you alive and on a path to health while at the same time a smile and a kind word. Imagine if you would, whistling Disney songs while waiting in the bathroom for your patient to have a bowel movement? Where do we breed wonderful humans like this? One of the hardest parts about recovery is wiping away your tears, pulling it together and getting to work. With a stroke no amount of medicine, or time will bring you all the way. It's these small, incremental, shitty steps towards being a regular human. Look at me, I don't smell like pee or wow, I moved my arm are significant victories. There is nothing that can adequately prepare you for that. I imagine it must be like watching your infant lift their head or take that first step, but that you have a fricking mortgage with that person.

I can't really explain how tired I am. How everything I do, a work meeting, disciplining my kids, a trip downstairs to do the laundry, a long drive, a short walk drive me to just want to collapse in a chair and stare at the television. I can also tell you I won't stop fucking doing it, give me a challenge and it will be done. There's nothing like talking to some of the top medical professionals in the world, and saying, "I'm really fatigued", and they're like "yeah, that happens, there's a lot of theories about it".

There ain't no crying in stroke recovery, will there is but it's just really a waste of time, I mean I guess it's cathartic and all. One of the weirder outcomes is just these sudden episodes. There are times that I just start crying, sometimes a thankful wail, a nod to the blessings that have been given me and other times just realizing that life is just out of rational control. A fear that it will happen again, a fear that I will not be able to be the man I need to be and often just a reflective sob about this exhausting journey. But mostly because life is kinda cool and I don't want to lose it.

I think part of this sadness is the feeling of being physically weak. Without a doubt I am pretty confident about my emotional, mental and spiritual strength, these are things that are ill defined however and most of us men have usually measured ourselves by our physical strength. When tested by my therapists, I fell in the "normal" range of physical strength and ability for a man my age. If you have ever met my boys, not one of them is normal, as my mother once called them, "your oversized friends". We were always very physical and that part has been a struggle even as a middle aged guy. This winter I was tested as I saw several high school students (one in particular) hassling a guy at the bus stop that was down on his luck, normally it's where I would have stood up for the guy but I actually felt small and threatened as at that point a quick shove would have put me to the ground. There was no eminent physical threat to the guy who was just minding his own business, but still it was a new reality for me. Thankfully I'm to the point where that's not happening again, but it is humbling.

Okay, sort of rambling there, kind of what they call "zaba, zaba, Nyal" except without the booze. Hoping to deal more later with the emotional part of this recovery. Thanks for listening. I may need an outline.

I'd like to thank the Academy

Lookin' at the devil, grinnin' at his gun
Fingers start shakin', I begin to run
Bullets start chasin', I begin to stop
We begin to wrestle I was on the top

I want to thank you falettinme be mice elf agin
Thank you falettinme be mice elf agin

Sly & The Family Stone

Thursday, September 7th, 2017 is one year after my stroke, what us crippled folk call a "strokeversery." I've written about this before, so it may be unintentionally repetitive of one of my other chapters, but give the brain damaged guy a break. As Elena, said to me, "don't have another stroke".

On this day, I really want to show gratitude for all those who have helped me to get to this point. People that visited me over and over, people that brought food to my house, send gifts, helped around the house, just an enormous amount of collective effort and love. I'd like to think I'd reciprocate, but let's not test that fact anyone.

Yesterday, September 10th, we put together a team and rode 22 miles and raised 5800 dollars for my alma mater, Spaulding Rehabilitation Hospital.

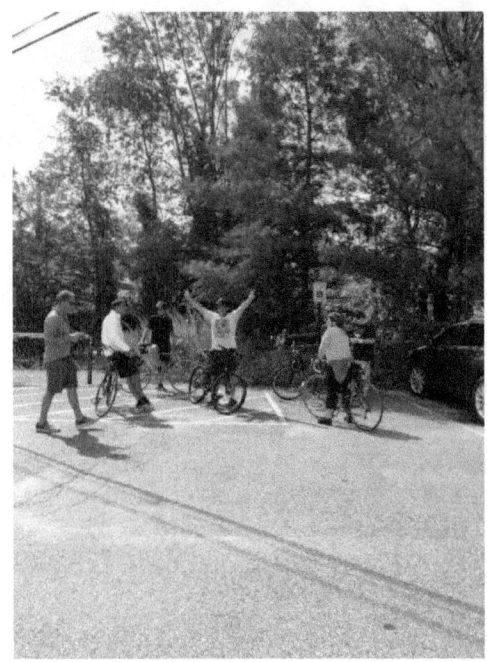

Half way point

A year ago my life was a shambles, I was defeated, I saw no way out, I think that the key was to stop using the word "I" too much. We are a collective species, our very long survival as homo sapiens has been built on our ability to think and work together. As a nation I think we sometime worship the power of individualism and hard work but that is just part of the equation, there are certainly times to be that "man in the arena" but there are essential chokepoints in life where individual action is the imperative, but who built that arena? Who keeps the arena running? I have had the gift over the past year by being supported by some of the most wonderful people anyone has had the fortune to come in contact with and never was I met with anything but the utmost support. All of you, led by supporter no. 1 Rebecca have had my back the entire time. When I was in the hospital it became a joke with the staff about how many visitors came (and I know now it's a pain in the ass to get there) and I knew other people got no one. But it's beyond the nice view of the Mystic, constantly folks have supported me in every way, doing stuff around my house, helping my wife, making food, watching the kids and just being patient with the sometimes-angry cripple. This support goes to my morale as well, going out of you way to spend time with me, talking, and reading my crazy shit. So, just let me say you're all awesome and you should take a bow.

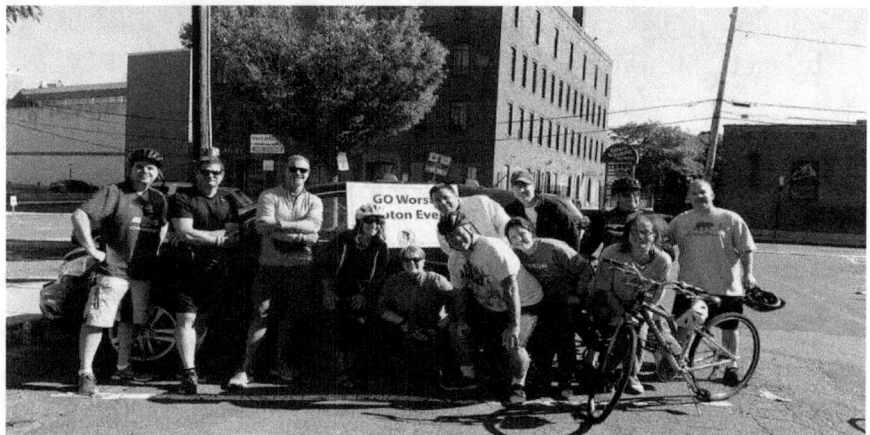

Yesterday, was super important to me, I actually didn't think I could do it physically and I was supernervous. A year ago to be honest I thought I was all done, cooked, fried, screwed and here we went clocking miles, sucking up asphalt and just enjoying a great day. we never know what tomorrow will bring but today was an awesome victory. thanks to all. Riding in to the ride with Clubba, I shared that fact, I had really no idea, I mean it's not a marathon but there are times I'm just exhausted walking to turn on the TV. To have this great group of friends by my side to share in this ride is an enormous part of my long-term recovery. A huge benchmark towards normalcy. I know I tend to be somewhat dramatic in people knowing about my recovery via social media, etc but I have to say it's really cool and important to have people rooting for me, praying and cheering me on, every effort has been noticed and y'all are building a karma and bbq bank with me. It felt a little selfish to be raising money for something that was about "me" and not about the kids, so I appreciate everyone who came out.

I am really overwhelmed and emotional this morning (and a little sore).We raised 6000 bucks, we had beers and briskets, although exhausted, I felt alive.

and again, THANKS to you and all your families, may we all lead blessed lives filled with joy and health together.

Remember When You Couldn't Smile?

I was so tired of being upset
Always wanting something I never could get
Life's an illusion, love is a dream
But I don't know what it is

Everybody's happy nowadays
Everybody's happy nowadays

Today, as I was sitting on my front stoop talking to my neighbor, she asked me "when did you see the light at the end of the tunnel?" I did talk about this in one chapter, but like most everything, I'm not sure that was true, you can try to predict a story but no one knows the outcome til the exit. I'm not sure the end of the tunnel is even there or if life is just really a series of tunnels, peaks and valleys, etc. I've made incredible advances in everything over the past year, physically, mentally, emotionally, spiritually, but yesterday when Reverend Dominic recognized my one-year anniversary in church, I can't say I didn't tear up, mostly out of being thankful but also out of a realization that I haven't reached the end of that proverbial tunnel yet. Today, presenting in front of a couple hundred people, I began to feel a little dizzy, probably like people feel once in a while, but then you get fearful, what's going on?, like life is a series of unpredictable events, I finished, walked off the stage, down the stairs, asking for a colleagues arm "just to be sure". I sat down for a few minutes and I was fine, but an indication that I'm not there yet. It sometimes makes me feel a little down at points, and fearful of an uncertain future, which in fact is the very definition of life.

There is a pretty good chance that this is the new normal. None of us will ever be a teenager or in our early twenties, with feeling of being indestructible and often self-destructive at the same time. But certainly, a traumatic brain injury has hastened the path of diminished ability. As it is said "youth is wasted on the young". Young people haven't developed the wisdom to appreciate what they have, an unbridled potential. There are struggles for sure, I was there, but the physicality of youth is but a distant memory for many of us struggling with physical recovery.

Recovery is a strange animal. There are many friends and family, probably in fact everyone that is in some stage of recovery. There are those that have survived the potential scourge of alcohol, tobacco and drugs. Those that suffered major illnesses and injuries certainly and those that are recovering from the loss of loved ones or even those that may have lost in love. I don't like the idea of commodifying or attaching value to levels of misery, we all meet life in different places.

Before the bike ride last week, I had one of my long conversations with clubba. I'm unsure if it's just the same conversation we've been having for the last thirty years plus, with frequent interruptions of time and distance as we live our lives together but apart. This is the nature of friendship, people you can share your hopes and dreams with, but also your dreads and fears, all of your ups and downs are just part of an ever-growing equation. I feel bad for people that can't have deep, shared friendships, because I don't think any kind of recovery is ever possible without it. When we were talking, he was telling about a point that I was talking so crazy and so depressed that he was about to "punch me in the side of the head". Like that bent armed f#ck thinks he could ever get around on me, no matter how crippled I was.

The point being, there is always a bottom and in every recovery, for every event there is always a time that you couldn't smile. I think it's important to remember and reflect on that. No matter how dark it is and how far that light is in the district, if you can smile, you are making progress. I remember the times that I couldn't, that the darker demons of life reigned victorious. There is something magical about a smile and a laugh when everything seems screwed up, somewhat of a cathartic rebellion against those that will knock you down. While all us existentialists know that life is fatal, we cannot let darkness get the last laugh.

We never know what life will bring us, challenges will always confront us and we have to rely on our inner strength (the self) and our outer strength (friends and family) to persevere. The key is knowing that you are not sure where the end of the tunnel is, but to always know you are moving in the right direction. And always remember, there was a time when you couldn't smile.

Mental Wealth

Radio, live transmission.
Radio, live transmission.

Listen to the silence, let it ring on.
Eyes, dark grey lenses frightened of the sun.
We would have a fine time living in the night,
Left to blind destruction,
Waiting for our sight.

And we would go on as though nothing was wrong.
And hide from these days we remained all alone.
Staying in the same place, just staying out the time.
Touching from a distance,
Further all the time.

Ian Curtis

Outside of maybe the stories of when I was first in the hospital, this is starting to be the most difficult chapter I've tried to write. Mostly because I'm going to get a lot of it wrong and perhaps even piss some people off. 90% of what I write is personal narrative, for the most part, a story of my own life, sprinkled in with some opinions and an occasional truth or factoid that I may have heard along the way. It's the laziest kind of writing, something Sally Polito at Cape Cod Community College and Roberta Roberts at Framingham State tried to knock out of my head, basically telling me, no one really cares what you think, they want facts. This is true of most academic writing and most of the writing I do for work, but here on the vast internets for my nearly dozens of readers, I can pretty much just type and carry on. This time it's a little more difficult as I'm trying to explain something I really don't understand, and that is mental health.

Most people don't really want to talk about mental health. It is something that is usually hidden and can sometimes be embarrassing. It's something that can affect your career, family and social life. I think over my lifetime we have become more upfront about mental health, seeing it more as a health issue rather than the concept of being being "crazy". Something that through therapy and pharma can be somewhat kept in control. Let me be clear, there are people that are still bat shit crazy, mental health be damned, but let's leave that there for now. About 4 more times I will own up to the fact that I don't know what I'm talking about, so if you are looking for a correct treatise on mental health to crib for your psychology paper, google on. I was a course short of a psych minor and probably took a couple more courses as a grad student and still have no idea about psychology.

I've had the benefit of moving up several social classes in my lifetime. From working class up to upper middle class. By income measures, our household is probably in the top quintile of income, with the requisite access to health care and education that comes with that. One thing that I have noticed is that mental health issues traverse across all these social classes. Certainly people who have our level of access to health care have much greater access to mental health care as well, but crazy really travels up and down American social classes, it's just easier to be a crazy rich person. However, in some ways, we are all aspiring to mental wealth, the idea that we are happy, unanxious, self-actualized, and generally comfortable in our own skin.

For this chapter, I did something unusual and solicited some help. Again, I don't really understand "mental illness". Certainly, I spent time of my life feeling sad, for a prolonged period of time, maybe even "depressed". Mostly listening to the Smiths, sipping Robitussin depressed. Most of the time I was my own worst enemy, self-medicating, making stupid decisions and mostly making things worse, but I think if you asked most people I was mostly a fairly balanced, glass is half full type of guy. For this chapter, I asked a couple of friends to come over for a couple beers and talk about mental health. The idea came from a conversation I had with one of my friends, Val, early on at my girls' school. I was talking about the emotional recovery challenges I was having early on, and she was amazingly insightful in reflecting on her own mental health experiences. They were completely different by the way, but really helped me to reflect.

As we sat at my dining room table for this extended conversation, Val was joined by her husband, Woody. Val and Woody are two of the wonderful people we have been lucky to run into as parents at our kids' school. Both are bright, articulate and generous folks, I think to an outsider, it would be like "why the hell are you depressed?"

I learned a lot. I understood why I was depressed, I had a major brain injury that tried to kill me. I still go to bed sometimes somewhat terrified that it's going to happen again. I would probably say I may have some sort of post-traumatic stress disorder although I don't want to say this when I have friends and family who have actual diagnoses after being in combat. It's hard to imagine these two being equal. But I still go into a mighty dark place from time to time. I had times of what they called "suicidal ideation" early on in the hospital, mostly due to the fact that my entire life had been dumped in the gutter and I was watched 24 hour a day at MGH for a couple days to prevent any attempts, as many of you have read it was about a dream I related to nurses there, I was never really suicidal and even then I don't know how someone who was paralyzed on one side of their body could do it. Nonetheless, I was assigned a psychologist once I was in rehab. I'm not a counselor type of guy, I'll talk about stuff to my friends and whatnot, but my entire thought in the times he was there was "how do I get this honkey out of my room?" (most of my philosophy is more George Jefferson, less Foucault)

Val talked openly about her depression. If not PTSD, I would describe my depression as episodic depression. I'm not sure if that's a thing or if I'm just making it up. It was a reaction to a specific event, a rational and emotional reaction as part of non-clinical depression, I was generally having a hard time dealing with the fact that I was facing an uncertain diagnosis which had completely turned my life upside down. This uncertainty spiraled me into frequent sobbing and tears and a general malaise that seemed unconquerable for a bit. Then I would watch Robocop, Michelle Obama on carpool karaoke or Marisol saying something silly and just laugh my ass off.

Clinical depression is an entirely different evil force, it's spirit animal is Donald Trump. I never really could understand, your life seems great, what's the problem. It's an entirely different thing to what I was experiencing. She described it in great detail, as a feeling you can't think or motivate yourself out of, sapped of energy, feeling dread, almost a physical hurt. A feeling that even if you're not suicidal, you just don't want to exist, clinical depression is not rational, you feel like you're losing your mind, and madness is setting in. She describes an inner monologue that is non-existent or less present, like being asleep, and feeling like the walking dead.

We all agreed that depression is a stupid word, it's too many things being described by one word, sort of the opposite of the trope around Eskimos and words for now. There certainly is the clinical, that is not necessarily attached to a specific event, which can vary from depressive episodes that are completely paralyzing to what Woody called dystimia or low-grade depression, a gnawing, persistent leech on your life. This spectrum or continuum can also manifest itself as irritability in the best of scenarios and in worse situations it is a form of madness, a storm in the brain. Val used William Styron's words (of course she did) as "darkness visible", an unwanted guest that you can't think out of your mind.

Again, there are not good definitions for depression writ large, it's just that clinical depression doesn't necessarily need to be triggered by a specific event.

For a stroke (or other) survivor I think it is important to reflect on mental health. In my case, I think my reaction as with many others was a normal reaction to a life changing event. There probably is still value for talk therapy or even drugs to assist in recovery. I was on Prozac for six months as part of an off-label use for brain recovery, I imagine the psychological effect were there as well. For those who have previous mental health issues, it is important to get "that stuff" as much as you can in check. Key pieces to recovery are hard work physically and a positive attitude. I think it is easy to confuse frustration and a longing for what used to be as depression for many of us that suffer from these non-clinical mental health maladies. There is a reluctance to face the fact that we are different than we were before our incidents, for better, for worse or for in between.

The day my Dad went to the Hospital

(This was written by my daughter Elena over a year after the event)

Siren's flashing as tears stream down my already tear soaked cheeks. My dad's stretcher gets pulled into an unfamiliar vehicle, blue suited people following him in.

One night, me and my sister, Marisol were watching tv. My dad called for me to come upstairs, but I didn't come up. A second later, he yelled "Elena come up here it's an emergency!"

"Coming!" I yelled as I dashed upstairs. When I entered his room, he was sitting on the floor next to his bed. He tells me to hand him the phone so he can call 911.After I hand him the phone I run to the bathroom and start bawling while screaming "I think I'm gonna puke!" He tells me to come back in and hands me the phone he says, "talk to Mama." When I take the phone into my trembling hands my mom tells me "go tell Christie to come and watch you and Marisol."

Next, I tell my sister to come with me to go get Christie. We run out the door, our bare feet pounding on the concrete street. When we come to the door we bang on it. When the door finally opens we tell Mike (Christie's husband) that we NEEDED Christie! When Christie comes downstairs I shout, "it's an emergency!"

"I'm coming, I'm coming" she says. As we walk briskly down the street the ambulance pulls up. My dad somehow walks down the stairs and is then brought to the ambulance by a few EMT's. I start crying some more as I watch the stretcher holding my dad being pulled into the ambulance. The EMT says to me he'll be okay."

Finally, after the ambulance left Christie said, "do you want a Kleenex?" since my eyes were teary and I kept sniffling. About an hour later my Uncle Rob showed up to get stuff for my mom and dad. Soon after, my Grandma Georgie showed up to take care of me and Marisol. We stayed up until about 10:00 watching *Chopped*. I called my mom again and it turned out that she was already coincidently at MGH visiting her friend.

As I lay in bed staring up at the ceiling, I think to myself "will he be okay?"

Cane and Able

Let me tell you the story of right hand-left hand. It's a tale of good and evil. Hate: it was with this hand that Cain iced his brother. Love: these five fingers, they go straight to the soul of man. The right hand: the hand of love. The story of life is this: static. One hand is always fighting the other hand, and the left hand is kicking much ass. I mean, it looks like the right hand — Love — is finished. But hold on, stop the presses; the right hand is coming back. Yeah, he got the left hand on the ropes now, that's right. Ooh, it's a devastating right and Hate is hurt. He's down. Left-Hand Hate KO-ed by Love. Radio Raheem (RIP)

Got some great response from Elena's entry, she really appreciated hearing everyone's kind words, hopefully we can have her write again, she has two different essay contests coming up, (one for VFW and one for MLK day) so I will try to share those with her adoring hordes. Also for those that are interested, I have copies of my book updated to include pretty much everything I've written other than the last few posts, so if you want a copy I have a bunch and they are also available for purchase on Amazon.

If you are an older person like me who grew up watching sports, you may remember Wide World of Sports. Before the proliferation of cable television and ESPN, Wide World of Sports was probably the only place outside of the Olympics where you could watch anything outside of the 4 major team sports, golf and tennis. But the thing that most of use probably remember is Jim McKay's intro which talked about the "thrill of victory and the agony of defeat".

15 months out, there are days that I still feel "the agony of defeat". Not that I think there are really bad days, but some aren't as good as others and ultimately through my brain trauma, I feel like I'm never going to be where I was or where I want to be. It took me a little while, but I now really get weirded out by the word "victim" in relationship to my incident. And I as most that are in recovery, really prefer the word "survivor". I think that it is a pretty important distinction, you aren't really the victim of a shipwreck, you're a survivor of a shipwreck. And the fact that you consider yourself as a survivor means that you have some agency in your own recovery.

Like that skier crashing in the beginning of Wide World of Sports, the feeling of defeat can be pretty consistent. This stroke has become an incredible, horrible part of my life story, my narrative if you would. I wake up in the morning with a headache and panic, thinking it is another stroke and not a simple clogged sinus or residual effects of a couple too many IPAs the night before. I continue to run like a toddler, and can't jump at all, still having some residual effects on the left side of my body as I try to recapture some youthful exuberance. The return of icy sidewalks and snow is also a reminder that my balance is not up to my former Nadia Comaneci standards. When I do work on my home projects, old lefty is not as precise as I need it to be. And of course, the worse part about it is the fatigue. One person on a stroke support group compared it to normal people having a 15-hour battery and stroke survivors having a 4 hour battery. 8-hour work days are exhausting and often end up with me, sitting in my easy chair after, trying to relax. A good night's sleep used to be enough to recharge, but that full recharge never seems to happen. Just so tired, all the time. There are theories for neuro-fatigue that I have heard; the most common one is that your brain rewiring itself (neuroplascity)take a lot of energy out of you, in my case it's the rest of my brain trying to take over for the part of my brain that died. That shit is just really hard for me to wrap my damaged mind around, although my body wasn't taken that day, a really important part had, and my annoyances today are a residual effect of that one traumatic event.

The chronicle of the agony of defeat is something we carry with us all the time, it is difficult to pull up that anchor. It is important for all survivors of all ordeal to understand the thrill of victory. Most of life is not really extreme highs and lows, yes, there is the occasional joy of say a wedding and the dread of a funeral but these are outliers. It is difficult to think about and enjoy everyday victories. I think my first victory is being alive, strokes kill a lot of people. Living of course, was an enormous victory and a smarter person than me may consider that victory to be the equivalence of a rebirth or restart and that every day from now on is a blessing, just gravy. I can't go that far and to be honest that despite this huge victory of living, I do feel cheated. Too young to be a cripple in recovery, was too healthy for this to happen and the requisite cry from those that are struck down, "why me" (apologies to Nancy Kerrigan)

I think also just general physical recovery has been a victory. Many people I meet have no idea I had a stroke and even people I know will often say "I can't believe how

much you recovered, you can't even tell you had a stroke."
I often say that I'm about 70% physically of where I was. I
can ride a bike, I can use power tools (well not
simultaneously), I can drive a car, go up and down stairs,
and haven't used a cane for several months. In fact, I think
most people that just meet me have no idea that some 14
months ago one side of my body was completely
paralyzed. It is difficult to explain what paralysis is like.
When you intentionally try to get your brain to make a
part of your body move and it just won't go anywhere. It is
incredibly terrifying. Recovering from this paralysis
happened in stages, the ability to stand in the early days
was an incredible event and through a lot of hard work,
eventually walking with a cane and then unaided. At
every point along the way, I felt defeated, I definitely tried,
somewhat successfully, to push that defeat down and
concentrate on the work at hand, as I have often written,
positivity is essential for success, the people I saw in rehab
who had given up had no real chance at recovery, the
harder you work and the more positive you are, inspires
those that work with you, the therapists, the nurses, your
family and friends to work even harder to support you in
your recovery. There are hiccups along the way, my
subluxation in my shoulder (dislocation) was insult to
injury. "Here asshole, you can move your arm now, but
I've separated the most important part." Every couple
steps forward, it would feel like you would have another
slip back.

There are even the smaller victories, things you never
think about. Being able to take care of your own hygiene.
Using the toilet without assistance, brushing your teeth,
showering are all really blessings, not having to use a

shower chair or assistive grab bars around the toilet is really fantastic. The ability to drive a car and just have the bus or lyft be an option rather than a requirement. The ability to go down and upstairs. For a long amount of time, I didn't get an opportunity to visit my workbench due to the vexing basement stairs.

I always like to think that the thrills of these victories will overcome the agonies of the defeats. However, it is a consistent battle in my mind and soul. On a daily basis I will feel really down and defeated, fearful of having another stroke and/or frustrated by the day to day struggle to get better. A lot of this frustration is due to the plateau effect. The changes and improvements become so small and immeasurable, that you don't put in the work and effort that needs to be done. Almost like a self-fulfilling prophecy, I know I have to work harder both in mind and body to improve. I think we would all do better if we learned to value our victories as much as we begrudge our defeats.

You're Gonna Fall Down

If I should fall from grace with god
Where no doctor can relieve me
If I'm buried 'neath the sod
But the angels won't receive me

Let me go, boys
Let me go, boys
Let me go down in the mud
Where the rivers all run dry-The Pogues

In the hospital for a long time, you gather a lot of wisdom from the people around you. Often wisdom is observed, and hopefully recorded in your addled brain like some cut rate betamax tape but joyfully sometimes it is quantified in words and sentences, an algorithm of letters designed to stick in your memory and fuel your soul.

One of my most memorable quotes (that I have stated in this tome before) came from my night nurse, Jill. There are dark times when you lie there alone in initial recovery, your visitors, of which I was blessed with many, have left and you are just left by yourself with occasional dropins from staff. Jill, with her positive attitude and brash, Boston girl OFD swagger would always be a highlight of my night and we would chat about random stuff as she went about her rounds. Early on when my entire left side was paralyzed, she would come in and tuck me in. Pulling a sheet and light blanket over my useless body. One night, I felt a little feeling in my foot and slowly moved my toes. A lot of time when you can't move, you sometimes imagine something or maybe gravity just doing what it does. I asked Jill if she could actually see my toes move, and she said yes. I responded, "fuck yeah" and she repeated "fuck yeah, imagine what you will do tomorrow." I know I've told this story before, but there is not a day or maybe even a couple of hours that I don't actually hear her voice in my ear. Imagine what you will do tomorrow, how in the living hell did she manage to say the most perfect statement at the right time. A gift from God, maybe? I am a praying man and it was an answer to a prayer. Those in recovery frequently make these pleas for assistance, hoping for a magical deity to make things right. But it don't roll like that, faith and prayer bring you the strength to work back, and it's hard to comprehend that.

But this this entry is really about another quote that really resonates with me. As I began to work back on walking and moving to walking with a cane in what is called close contact, I had a substitute physical therapist (PT), I've spoken much about Molly, my regular PT that saved my life, but there were a series of people who dove into help along the way. At this session, my wife happened to be there, as I walked along slowly, half leaning on my PT, the PT said to me, "you're gonna fall down, just fall down the right way". In more detail she said most of fall injuries happen as people are going downstairs, falling upstairs is usually not a problem. Understanding you are going to fall down is critical in life. I have been lucky in this effect in literally falling down, one incident in public at a Tuskegee airman presentation where my knee collapsed and I fell to the ground in front of my daughter and about 300 other people, physically I was fine, but emotionally it can take a toll.

But what is more important to think about is the more metaphorical falling down. 16 months out, with a huge amount of recovery, I am still falling down. It is exhausting to recover. Recently my girls have taken up basketball, having never played, we went down to the Y courts to work on some fundamentals. I loved basketball, during some of my shitty times as a younger man, it was a place where everything bad disappeared. Where I could hang around with my friends, play ball and bust on each other. Cold, hot, whatever we were out on that blacktop. My girls have graduated to nice, flat wood floors with climate control, which is pretty sweet. I took that ball in my hand, dribbled a bit, trying to get that old flavor, that feeling of moving around the court, taking some shots, chasing my inevitable missed shot, etc. But I fell down, not literally, I kept my feet but I was clumsy, missing layups and unable to jump enough to get off a decent shot or chase down the misses. It was frustrating. Now the positive person in me should be thankful to be out there in the first place, the joy of playing with your kids, enjoying more days above ground. It hurts though, I'm not who I was, I've fallen down. I can't stop thinking about my inability to move fluidly, when I should be focusing on my ability to move at all.

Life is a series of struggles. For the first time in a long time in my life, I struggle with my mental health around maintaining a positive attitude. There are times when I randomly feel sad and teary and most of all tired. Mostly I live a good life, filled with family and friends, Ups and downs that tend to regress towards the mean. Again, this is somewhat metaphorical. I fall down. I've changed. My body still will not do what I want it today, but then again, imagine what I will do tomorrow.

Curses and Blessings

I write this as I take a personal day after the Patriots loss in Superbowl 52, I think years of Red Sox futility in our youth always felt as cursed, but we have definitely been blessed in this 21st century in Boston sports. This is the most simplistic way to looking at a blessing and curse. Measurable to a degree and fairly easy to understand albeit a completely false dichotomy, neither blessing or curses in these cases are built on an extraordinary force but a culmination of talent acquired and timing of other teams acquiring talent. (both on-field/court and off). I think as fans we want to consider ourselves part of these ups and downs, but for the most part we are just knowledgeable observers. I have no idea why I started this that way, but just felt a need to comment on the news of the day.

On Wednesday, I will be 17 months "post-stroke". It's weird to write "post" as it's not like something that has gone away, like the loss of a Superbowl or Valentine's Day or something. It's something that those of us who are in recovery carry forever. Over these 17 months, I have battled between the thoughts of whether I am blessed or cursed. Intellectually, I know that it is hard to conceive of blessings and curses in an existential sense, in the same way that one may think of sorcery. A stroke is a biological malfunction, in my case, some type of clot ending up in my brain and permanently damaging a portion of it, and again in my case causing a temporary inability to use the left side of my body and maybe a permanent mild disability to use that side. That's the curse I guess, what in bronze age times (and with some people now) would be consider a "smiting" from above. The blessing of course is that I survived and as you have seen from these writings was met with an incredible outpouring of love and support and level of medical care that would seem impossible even for the most privileged and wealthy of people.

Stroke Recovery

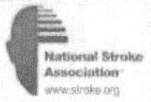

National Stroke
Association
www.stroke.org

- 10% of stroke survivors recover almost completely

- 25% recover with minor impairments

- 40% experience moderate to severe impairments requiring special care

- 10% require care within either a skilled-care or other long-term care facility

- 15% die shortly after the stroke

As you can see above, the majority of people are not as "blessed" as I am. These numbers are terrifying, in fact in a study in the Netherlands, only 3 of 5 people under 50 who had a stroke were alive in five years. Part of my relative success was my age, while there are certainly quite a few people who have strokes in their forties, it is far from the majority, and also many stroke survivors (and non-survivors) suffered from co-morbidities such as diabetes, heart disease and other chronic diseases that affected their function. I had been generally "blessed" with good health before this event. Also having really fast access to health care including a $37,000 clot busting drug.

In the graphic above, I see myself in category 2 at this point with maybe a future potential of reaching level 1. My biggest complaints tend to be around neurofatigue, which is really being tired for no specific reason, but my brain works too hard as it continues to re-wire itself to make up for the damaged part of my brain (or so the theory goes), some left side weakness (grip for one, and sometimes on stairs) and some weird lack of recalling particular words I am looking for (which I attribute to said neuro-fatigue). I also am pretty slow when it comes to running, I'm re-learning how to swim (I can dog paddle and tread water, I'm just working of freestyle and speed) and a virtual inability to jump. (which is probably one of the oddest of them all). On the positive side, I've been shooting baskets with the girls, walk at my usual 4 mph pace (I remember .5 mph being a goal in rehab), can ride a bike well, use power tools, ladders, drive a car, work full time, etc. When tested in March, I tested within average levels for a man my age.

So blessed or cursed. I think for most survivors, there is some cognitive dissonance. Your head swimming as you try to figure out what just happened and why it would happen to you. However, these are somewhat meaningless labels that can distract from recovery at some points. The only thing that may be as frustrating as people feeling sorry for me are those that call me "lucky". Lucky, what the fuck are you talking about, at a time where most dads with kids my age were out running around with their kids, I was in a fucking wheel chair smelling of drops of urine and wondering if I would ever walk again. Not sure how lucky that is, but then again, I understand, even when I was in the hospital, I saw those that would fit the label of cursed, those with severe cognitive dysfunction, those that didn't seem to be making any progress, but more so those that had a really negative attitude and those who had no one in their corner, no visitors, no Becky to make their long cruel days a little brighter, no children to come and harass them, because in those latter people you found little light to cut through the darkness. As a "norm" today, it is much easier to see the blessings that I had even in my darkest days as a "crip." And even as I see those whose recovery trajectories are much slower than mine, I can see what people see as blessings. I belong to a stroke recovery group on Facebook where you can really see the struggles that people go through over years and years of recovery. From time to time I participate in a stroke recovery group at Spaulding, but it is really difficult, my recovery has been so good (relatively) that I sometimes struggle with the fact that people who continue to suffer, not only physically, but cognitively for years. These are the folks that tend to go to these meetings, folks that are struggling but have positive attitudes towards life, brought by doting caregivers and family (caregivers in all of this are the true blessing) I don't think a lot of them even years after their stroke could even imagine playing 1 on 2 in basketball against their 11-year-old daughter and her friend or riding a bike 22 miles. At the same time, I'm not sure I'll ever lace up those sneakers and get in a game with adults again, not sure if I could jump for a rebound or come off a pick.

Sometimes with our kids to avoid 2-hour blow by blow recaps of their days, we ask them to give us a rose and a thorn, a rose being a good thing, a thorn something that was not so good. Two things that are much different. I guess if blessings and curses do exist, they are not absolutes. For the most part I think they are inaccurate descriptors. The human need to quantify something that is inexplicable and likely does not exist. In some ways, it is the equivalent of trying to figure out how Santa gets billions of presents produced, on a sled and delivered to all of the world's Christian children in 24 hours.

The Hindus have a word called karma. The way I understand it is that your future lives are built upon their actions in a previous existence. While I can't pretend to understand, comprehend or believe this, I imagine that most of us like to think the previous actions in our lives affect those later in our lives and in some ways having a stroke is a rebirth of sorts, a completely life changing event. Maybe some of these blessings were built off my own life and efforts to date. I'd like to think this is somewhat true, that I would have some agency in my own future and not just be an unwilling participant on a health nantucket sleigh ride. But mostly because it is difficult in general to cede control to an unseen and unknown force thought to be a blessing or curse.

So, I guess it's mostly about being in control. Whether it's good or bad being able to steer your own direction. After a lifetime of self-sufficiency it is difficult to surrender to the fates.

A Clean Bill of Health

Just a short, boring entry that is really more of a personal health update vis a vis, some deep philosophical shit. From the beginning of this story, I have tried to make sure people understand a bunch of things as they read this. Perhaps the most important is, don't take any medical advice from me. (except the image directly below) I don't really know much about the actual physiology of a stroke and obviously since I had one, you probably shouldn't listen to anything I have to say about preventing one. That being said, one thing I don't think I've ever been really emphatic about is the importance of getting medical care as fast as possible for you or your loved ones who may be having a stroke. In my entire time meeting dozens of people in the hospital who had strokes, only one person, who was an emergency room nurse, had any idea what the hell was going on.

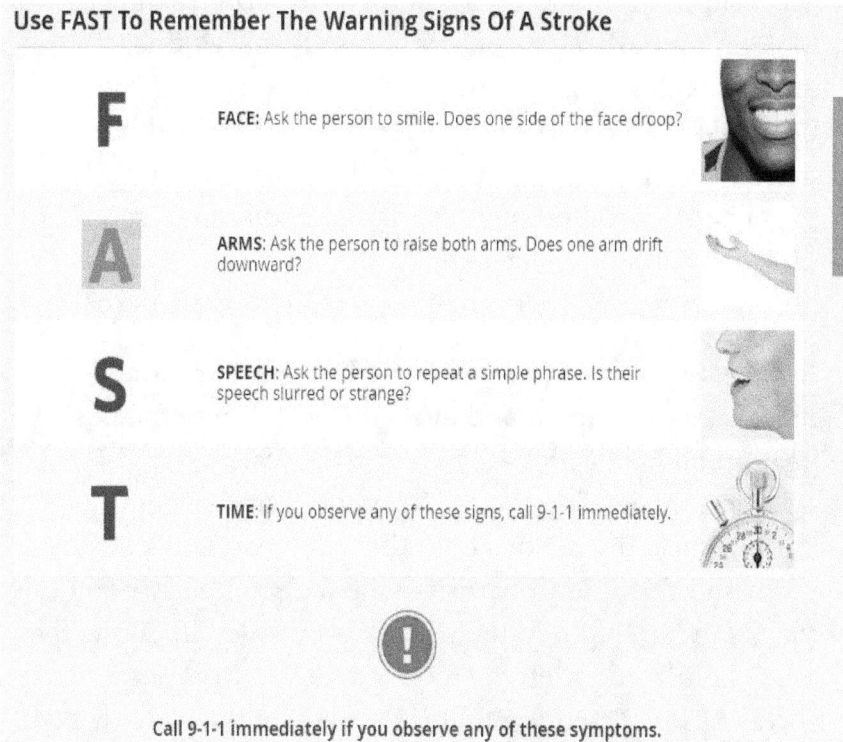

Use FAST To Remember The Warning Signs Of A Stroke

F — **FACE:** Ask the person to smile. Does one side of the face droop?

A — **ARMS:** Ask the person to raise both arms. Does one arm drift downward?

S — **SPEECH:** Ask the person to repeat a simple phrase. Is their speech slurred or strange?

T — **TIME:** If you observe any of these signs, call 9-1-1 immediately.

Call 9-1-1 immediately if you observe any of these symptoms.

These things are simple, and call 9–1–1, they'll get you there faster, get you in the door and let the right people know you're coming, minutes matter, your brain cells are dying, deprived of oxygen, and there are specific drugs (tPA for one) that can help to break those clots if you get to the hospital in time. (in the case of an ischemic stroke) I can't imagine how bad things could have been without the blessings of Melrose FD, Melrose-Wakefield Hospital and MGH that first day.

On Friday, I had my annual physical. One of the things I avoided over the years were these annual physicals, what I am sad to say (and my doc never has said) I often wonder if I could have prevented said stroke by regular medical appointments, blood pressure meds and pretty much looking for early signs of any issues. But I felt fine, I always said, lose 20 pounds and I'd be a fricking Olympian. When I was younger and had no health care, there was an excuse, regular medical care can be really expensive when you have to make a choice between rent or tuition or food or seeing a doctor, but now I (and most nearly everyone in Massachusetts really have no excuse).

I still hate going to the even after I've been prodded, medicated, therapied and everything else over the past year and a half. I prepare myself to be lectured at, questioned like Goering at Nuremburg and generally chastised for my actions over the past year. Unlike the daily and then monthly visits with a doctor early on, these visits are not that frequent. The stress builds up in me the week before and then the requisite blood work. In this case it was lipids. The thing that is interesting now is how fast you can get the results. I got the results, and everything was great but this one thing, triglycerides. My triglycerides were way above normal and knew this a couple days before the actual appointment.

My primary care provider is awesome, a woman probably in her late thirties, who is a mom of young kids. (this makes a difference to me, kids are exhausting and it's good to have someone that understands that) She looks at health holistically the balance of head and body, is really up on the new research, really loves data and is intellectually curious. Early on, when I just got out of the hospital (which is the first time I met this PCP, I know right) I met her, we had a great conversation, she was strangely comforting although at that first visit although she did say to me, "there are going to some times when you feel like you may be having a stroke again, definitely go through the protocols (FAST protocols), but chances are you aren't having a stroke, it's just a weird part of your brain rewiring." Wow, thanks, doc, that's fucking comforting.

So, at the visit the first thing I brought up was the lipid data. "Oh, I think it looks great". I ask her about the triglycerides, and she was like, "oh, the range you were looking at were for fasting, nobody who ate anything is going to have those numbers". So great, my panic was for naught. In fact, that particular count is not really related to cardiovascular health. "I told you last time, if you were ever wondering about anything, just give me a call". In fact, I had made an appointment with her a few months ago concerned about rapid pulse, her nurse had also told me "you don't have to be on your death bed to make an appointment." These are things that despite all the care I've had in the last 18 months are still hard to understand, you have help out there when you need it.

Physicals are weird because you talk about shit that you wouldn't talk about with anyone else, "do you have problems urinating, have you noticed blood in your stool, and other not for prime-time discussions. Mostly when you go to the doc, you want to get out there as quickly as possible with solutions and observations that your mom may have; you should drink less, you should exercise more, you could lose some weight, why don't you bring my grandkids to visit me and things of that ilk.

Our conversation was long, we started out talking about predictive analytics, which is actually one of my work projects and just a pretty long data conversation and about how controlling numbers, particularly blood pressure just has an enormous effect on secondary prevention. Secondary prevention is basically, you let that damn horse out of the barn, now fix that damn door. Medication for the rest of my life is a part of this, but certainly lifestyle changes can help. Lose weight, less stress, drink water, exercise can all help in the control of blood pressure but some of it is hereditary. There are some people who won the blood pressure lottery, who you would not imagine. She gave me a series of very achievable goals and the stress of the visit soon disappeared.

So essentially, I was given a clean bill of health. A little roadmap to my continued recovery. It is a long journey, I'm not where I want to be yet, I'm tired, I misstep, I occasionally lose my temper (usually just to myself) but my life has really been given back to me. It's not a total George Bailey feeling, I guess; the whole stroke thing still pisses me off and scares the crap out of me, but away I go, papa, husband, human, Nyal.

Prologue
(Ok, the initial prologue)

No, recovery has not come to an end. I had a couple initial goals when I was in the hospital, one was to go to my daughter's birthday party in early October, the second is to cook a Thanksgiving dinner like we are all used to. Even by my standards our Thanksgiving meal is ridiculous. We just go out of the way to make enough food and drink to feed an army. This year will have the additional assistance of clubba and uncle Scott to help us deliver this bounty. It is indicative of the past few months, work hard and have other people support you and you'll be successful. A thunderbolt struck me down temporarily but I'm picking myself off the floor and moving forward. It sucks, sometimes I can't deal with it, but it's reality and you live and try to be further successful in everything you do. Returning to work and the holidays will be challenging but it is incredibly large part of my happiness and well-being. I hope to write more and add to these volumes. In a couple of months, I hope to be driving and being able to go to Spaulding and volunteer some of my time. I hope my day-to-day gets easier and that my life becomes fuller even though is quite full right now. I know I have done this throughout these volumes but the best of thanks and love to all my family and friends who have been there for me especially my wife. I would also like to thank Karyn Sultan Hendricks for assistance in editing parts of this first edition, all mistakes still remain my own. Karyn was a good friend of my mom and dad and lived with us when I was kid, she was always super good to us and it was nice to reconnect via Facebook and for her to assist me in this effort. Life is a crazy quilt, a function of space and time, all of your efforts are for not without the love and consideration of others.

(Revisited November 2017)

A year after starting this project and mostly posting it on medium.com, I decided to do a second edition, you know for the holidays, because everyone likes to read about stroke recovery around the yule log. It's a continuing effort, I just got back from the docs this afternoon, heart is in good shape, clean ECG, my heart just likes to move a little faster than others. My life is not totally obsessed with doc's, med's, therapists and tests, it's mostly normally although to probably a different beat than most people. I drive, I do work around the house, parent, volunteer and work excessive hours like many of my generation. Sometimes the left leg doesn't want to come along as fast and I'm not as facile with my left hand on projects than I once was, but not that bad. I do lay awake sometimes in fear and trepidation of the unknown, but who's to say everyone isn't doing that. I do want to challenge myself more physically in the new year but also want to challenge myself and you dear reader in the new year in a different plane. Maybe we can all learn to be kinder, to understand the very nature of modern humanity is that we are all coming from different places and attitudes, with unseen struggles as we try to navigate life.

Cripple: An Epilogue (August 2018)

I was hoping we'd make real progress -
But it seems we have lost the power
Any tiny step of advancement
Is like a raindrop falling into the ocean -
We're running on the spot — always have — always will?
We're just the next generation of the emotionally crippled.
Though we keep piling up the building blocks
The structure never seems to get any higher
Because we keep kicking out the foundations
And stand useless while our lives fall down.
I believe in life — and I believe in love

But the world in which I live in — keeps trying to prove me wrong.

Paul Weller

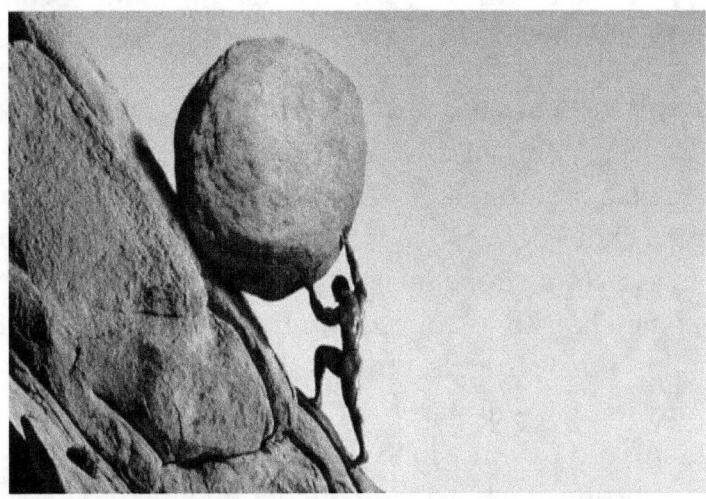

It is the beginning of July of 2018, my writing has got much more infrequent as to be honest there are not many tales to tell. There is just the day to day of middle aged employed dad living, hustling around and just trying to take care of business with little time to really be reflective. I imagine we all suffer (or in some cases benefit) from that, the lack of time to really spend times in our own heads. If you are reading this in my book, this is the epilogue, that is sort of a closing reflection as I add in some unpublished chapters and go towards another edition. I may pop into the blog on occasion with updates.

Early on, I spent a lot more time writing. Sometimes as a way to escape my daily fears but some put on toughness, sometimes to celebrate small victories but overall to chronicle my recovery for myself and others.

Recovery, as I have frequented opined is an odd beast, as liberating as it is frustrating. Simultaneously having a profound state of deep sadness for what you have lost along with the intense happiness of having another chance. As with all forms of recovery it is incredibly frustrating.

In many ways I'm unsure if I will ever completely recover, in fact as I age I'm not even sure what the baseline is. Sewing on a button today was something I could not have dreamed about doing 18 months ago but at the same time my old eyes (not stroke related) and left-hand dexterity (still somewhat stroke related extremely fine motor skills) made this a real struggle. On occasion when I get really tired, my left leg will start to drag, which was probably best displayed by our trip to Puerto Rico, where 16th century fortification designs were not intended for somewhat out of shape, middle aged stroke survivors. Mostly, however, it is the unrelenting fatigue and exhaustion. I am not hopeful that this will subside, and it has definitely hampered my fitness goals and maybe even some professional and personal goals as well. I have not been a good sleeper for a long time, but now even with what would be a good night of sleep for me, generally I'm still exhausted most of the day, not just tired but often a nearly crippling fatigue that is very hard to explain.

Cripple is a weird word. From Day 1 in the hospital I feared I'd never walk or function like a human being again. It's not like you cut your finger and you know it's eventually going to heal, like it has a hundred times in your life. The inability to even move a finger or toe is completely terrifying. As far as most people with traumatic brain injuries go, I had a pretty expedited recovery trajectory but those first eight weeks was the most traumatic time of my life. Those first couple weeks in rehab, I marveled at those who could walk with little assistance in the support group, going so far as to create my binary "crips" and "norms" grouping.

I guess in most cases, people would consider me to be a "norm" now, but in my heart of hearts, I'm a cripple. Whether it just be the extreme physical, emotional and spiritual teardown that was caused by the trauma or just an inability to do everything my brain wants me to do. (other than the bitch trying to kill me) There are certainly people who are a lot worse off than me, even after a long time. I've just gone to a couple post-release stroke support groups and most people who attend those meetings have a high level of disability, often physical, including many in wheelchairs five to ten years out and others with mental or speech issues or other co-morbidities (usually heart or breathing issues). It is very difficult to see a person who used to be an architect or a nurse struggle to play the simplest game. At the same time, the alternative, death, for most of us is probably much worse. So in most accounts, I am blessed.

It doesn't stop me from being cranky, depressed and frustrated. As with many traumatic one time events, we look at the sky and puzzle, "Lord, why me?" or just more a "what the fuck", depending on your theological outlook, I tend to do both. Some days, just getting through a regular day is a struggle, even in an office job that isn't physically challenging. My patience isn't what it used to be and I become much more easily frustrated. But I'm alive and kicking, I do find joy in life, in family, in friends, in my garden, in a way that I cried like a little baby about in Spaulding Rehab.

Someone told me a story about another stroke patient who also more recently spent a month in Spaulding. She didn't remember the names of anyone who worked on the floor. That just astonished me, I think of these people every day, and probably will until my last breath. I came to think there are two different ways to approach a miserable health situation. One, be miserable and know that the whole world is pulling for you or be miserable and think the whole world is against you. The latter is a formula for destruction.

Life is not linear, we use chronology to try to make sense of it, but that is just to frame our understanding. A recent visit to a support group reminded me of people, who have had a lot more time on their side to recover but still are in wheelchairs, with walkers or have severe speech abnormalities. I had some guilt about my own pretty good recovery, even as I still struggle to be who I was physically.

So maybe for the rest of my life, I will consider myself a "cripple". With stroke survivor being as important part of my identity as father, son, uncle, husband, etc. It is not a badge of honor, not even necessarily a ball and chain or a Sisyphean sphere but as important as any gender or racial ethnic or positional authority I may have. But in a sense, we are all survivors.

Nyal Fuentes, August 2018

Thank you for reading,

Nyal Fuentes

Melrose, Massachusetts